100 Questions About Breastfeeding

Karin Cadwell, PhD, RN, FAAN, IBCLC, RLC

Cindy Turner-Maffei, MA, IBCLC, RLC

Anna Cadwell Blair, PhD, CLC

JONES AND BARTLETT PUBLISHERS
Sudbury, Massachusetts
BOSTON   TORONTO   LONDON   SINGAPORE

World Headquarters
Jones and Bartlett Publishers
40 Tall Pine Drive
Sudbury, MA 01776
978-443-5000
info@jbpub.com
www.jbpub.com

Jones and Bartlett Publishers
Canada
6339 Ormindale Way
Mississauga, Ontario L5V 1J2
Canada

Jones and Bartlett Publishers
International
Barb House, Barb Mews
London W6 7PA
United Kingdom

Jones and Bartlett's books and products are available through most bookstores and online book-sellers. To contact Jones and Bartlett Publishers directly, call 800-832-0034, fax 978-443-8000, or visit our website www.jbpub.com.

Substantial discounts on bulk quantities of Jones and Bartlett's publications are available to cor-porations, professional associations, and other qualified organizations. For details and specific discount information, contact the special sales department at Jones and Bartlett via the above contact information or send an email to specialsales@jbpub.com.

The authors, editor, and publisher have made every effort to provide accurate information. However, they are not responsible for errors, omissions, or for any outcomes related to the use of the contents of this book and take no responsibility for the use of the products and procedures described. Treatments and side effects described in this book may not be applicable to all people; likewise, some people may require a dose or experience a side effect that is not described herein. Drugs and medical devices are discussed that may have limited availability controlled by the Food and Drug Administration (FDA) for use only in a research study or clinical trial. Research, clinical practice, and government regulations often change the accepted standard in this field. When consideration is being given to use of any drug in the clinical setting, the health care provider or reader is responsible for determining FDA status of the drug, reading the package insert, and reviewing prescribing information for the most up-to-date recommendations on dose, precautions, and contraindications, and determining the appropriate usage for the product. This is especially important in the case of drugs that are new or seldom used.

Production Credits
Executive Editor: Kevin Sullivan
Acquisitions Editor: Emily Ekle
Associate Editor: Amy Sibley
Editorial Assistant: Patricia Donnelly
Production Director: Amy Rose
Associate Production Editor: Wendy Swanson
Senior Marketing Manager: Katrina Gosek
Associate Marketing Manager: Rebecca Wasley
Manufacturing and Inventory Control Supervisor: Amy Bacus
Composition: Auburn Associates, Inc.
Cover Design: Jonathan Ayotte
Cover Image: © Vladimir Melnik/ShutterStock, Inc.
Printing and Binding: Malloy, Inc.
Cover Printing: Malloy, Inc.

Library of Congress Cataloging-in-Publication Data
Cadwell, Karin.
    100 questions and answers about breastfeeding / Karin Cadwell, Cindy Turner-Maffei,
Anna Cadwell Blair.
        p. cm.
    Includes index.
    ISBN-13: 978-0-7637-5183-8 (pbk. : alk. paper)
    ISBN-10: 0-7637-5183-9 (pbk. : alk. paper)   1. Breastfeeding—Miscellanea.   2. Breastfeeding—
Popular works.   I. Turner-Maffei, Cindy.   II. Blair, Anna Cadwell. III. Title.   IV. Title: One
hundred questions and answers about breastfeeding.
    RJ216.C22 2008
    649'.33—dc22

2007034035

6048
Printed in the United States of America
11 10 09 08 07   10 9 8 7 6 5 4 3 2 1

Contents

As a doctor who delivers babies, I thought that I understood, from taking care of my patients as they become parents, how incredible it is to have a child. But I truly did not understand the gift of parenthood until I myself became a mother (three times). As you embark on this wonderful journey, whether for the first time or the tenth, as a patient or as a healthcare provider, decision-making begins early. It goes without saying that we are all interested in maximizing the health and safety of mothers and children. Therefore, breastfeeding is the obvious choice for a child given its astounding number of significant health benefits, both short- and long-term, for both moms and kids.

And yet it's not always that easy, is it? There are still many barriers to breastfeeding, ranging from practical to societal. Mothers may have difficulty getting the specific medical help that they need at a particularly vulnerable point in their lives immediately after a baby is born. As a savvy patient of mine once commented, "You know, they don't have bottle feeding classes, do they?" More broadly, family, employers, and/or the general public may not wholeheartedly support a mother's decision to breastfeed.

This book is a very valuable source of information about breastfeeding, whether you are trying to decide what and how to feed your child or working out some of the details of prolonged nursing or something in between. Its simple, user-friendly format provides concise, practical answers to the questions that all parents have about breastfeeding their children. The questions are very relevant; the responses are thorough yet succinct, evidence based but also easy for tired new parents to understand. It is very exciting to have such a tremendous resource from an esteemed group of breastfeeding experts in this clear, easy-to-use format. If you choose to breastfeed your child, I am certain that this book can help you to achieve that goal.

I am an academic family physician with a maternal-child health practice that includes obstetrics, as well as a lactation consultant and the working mother of three breastfed children. I would recommend this book as a valuable breastfeeding resource to my colleagues, my patients, my medical students, and my friends.

Julie S. Taylor, MD, MSc, IBCLC
Associate Professor of Family Medicine
The Warren Alpert Medical School of
   Brown University
Memorial Hospital of Rhode Island
Pawtucket, Rhode Island

Acknowledgments

The authors are grateful to the many mothers who have shared with us their breastfeeding questions, concerns, successes, and struggles. Without this rich, shared "herstory," a book such as this would not be as true to the lived experience of breastfeeding. As we wrote this book, we remembered many of the mothers, babies, and families that we have had the honor of serving in our combined 70+ years of working in the field of breastfeeding. The questions in this book were generated from a review of the telephone logs of our breastfeeding warmline, which has been in existence for more than 10 years, as well as questions raised in our breastfeeding support groups and consults at the Healthy Children Project, Center for Breastfeeding, in East Sandwich, Massachusetts.

We wish to particularly thank our colleagues at the Center for Breastfeeding, particularly Zoë-Maja McInerney; the mothering experts from our weekly nursing mothers' support group and classes who generously reviewed the manuscript: Melissa Russell, Ellen Savage, and Sally Tabor; to our esteemed colleagues Roshann Hooshmand, MD and Julie Taylor, MD for making time to review the manuscript; and to all of our babies, children, families, and friends for providing us and our reviewers with time to read and write.

We also thank our talented illustrator Doreen for the beautiful art that illuminates this book.

Finally, this book is dedicated to *you*, the reader, with our very best wishes!

PART ONE

Choosing Breastfeeding

Is breastfeeding that much better than formula?

Should every woman breastfeed?

Can every baby breastfeed?

More ...

1. Everyone seems to be breastfeeding these days. What's going on?

You're right! Breastfeeding increased in popularity in the early 1970s after a decline of several decades, and the trend of more and more mothers choosing to breastfeed continues today. Along with that trend, many hospitals, birth centers, and healthcare providers have improved the help and support they offer to new mothers. Peer counselors, volunteer breastfeeding helpers, and breastfeeding care providers provide breastfeeding support and information as well.

When families are asked about why they chose to breastfeed, they give a variety of reasons, including the possible health problems that come with feeding **formula**, the price of formula, ecologic worries, and convenience.

Healthcare providers encourage women to breastfeed because of the growing list of negative health outcomes associated with not breastfeeding. Not only is a baby healthiest *while* being breastfed, but a child who is breastfed experiences fewer chronic diseases in the future, as well.

A 2007 US government report concluded that for babies in countries like the United States, being breastfed was associated with a reduced risk of ear infections, **gastrointestinal** problems, severe lower respiratory tract infections, skin problems caused by **allergy** (such as **eczema**), childhood **asthma**, childhood obesity, **type 1 (insulin-dependent)** and **type 2 (non-insulin-dependent) diabetes**, childhood leukemia, sudden infant death syndrome (SIDS), and necrotizing enterocolitis (NEC), a

Formula

a food made from cow's milk or soy milk that has been chemically altered to make it appropriate for the nutrition of human babies

Gastrointestinal

having to do with the stomach and intestinal tract

Allergy

an abnormal reaction to a protein that is eaten, inhaled, or otherwise encountered

Eczema

a noncontagious skin inflammation, characterized chiefly by redness, itching, and the outbreak of lesions that may become encrusted and scaly

Asthma

an inflammation or swelling of the airway, leading to breathing difficulty, wheezing, and coughing

Choosing Breastfeeding

3

Type 1 diabetes

a chronic illness caused by insufficient production of insulin and resulting in abnormal metabolism of carbohydrates, fats, and proteins; symptoms include increased sugar levels in the blood and urine, excessive thirst, frequent urination, and unexplained weight loss; this disease is treated with insulin and is also called "insulin-dependent diabetes mellitus"

Type 2 diabetes

a milder form of diabetes that typically appears first in adulthood and is associated with obesity and an inactive lifestyle; this disease often has no symptoms, is usually diagnosed by tests that indicate glucose intolerance, and is treated with changes in diet, exercise, and medications; it is also called "non-insulin-dependent diabetes mellitus"

severe and often fatal intestinal problem usually associated with babies born prematurely.[1]

For the mother, having breastfed was associated with a reduced risk of type 2 (non-insulin-dependent) diabetes. A woman who has breastfed also has a reduced risk of breast cancer and ovarian cancer. According to the same US government study, women who breastfed for a short time or did not breastfeed at all had a greater chance of postpartum depression compared to women who breastfed longer.

The cost of formula has been going up and up. It now costs a thousand dollars or more for formula during the 1st year of a baby's life. The exact amount depends on whether a family chooses a store brand or a more expensive name brand. This is one of the reasons families choose to breastfeed—they can use the money to buy other things!

Formula-fed babies have higher healthcare costs, too. They require more prescriptions, more hospital care, and other additional costs associated with sick baby health care. Parents of breastfed babies lose fewer days of work because their babies are sick less often.

In the past century women chose breastfeeding because they didn't have enough money to buy formula. Today movie stars and professional women who could afford to buy formula are breastfeeding because they know it's best for their baby and themselves.

As people become more and more conscious of how their choices impact the world, many families choose to

---

[1]Tufts-New England Medical Center Evidence-Based Practice Center. (2007). *Breastfeeding and maternal and infant health outcomes in developed countries*. Rockville, MD: Agency for Healthcare Research and Quality.

breastfeed for ecologic reasons. An enormous amount of energy, more than 100 billion BTUs a year, is used to prepare, package, and transport infant formula. The food ingredients that are used to manufacture formula could be used to feed hungry older children and adults.

Mothers also find breastfeeding easy—you can just take your baby and go out. There is nothing to buy, nothing to get ready.

Jenny couldn't decide whether to breastfeed. All the reasons she was given seemed important, but she still found making the decision difficult. She asked a lot of questions and read several books. Then the baby's father said to her, "You hate to even carry a purse. My pockets are always full of your stuff! If you breastfeed, you will always have plenty of milk available and at the right temperature. You can put a diaper in your pocket and go!" Jenny decided that breastfeeding was right for her, and it was.

Mothers also describe the special relationship they have with their baby as a reason to breastfeed.

Tiffiny didn't have any friends or family members who had breastfed their babies, but the nurse at the prenatal clinic encouraged her to think about breastfeeding. She did, and weeks later, when the nurse asked Tiffiny about why breastfeeding might be a good choice for her, Tiffiny said, "If I breastfeed, everyone will know I'm the mother. Only I can breastfeed my baby. That will make me special to her."

Mothers give plenty of non-health-related reasons to breastfeed, such as "breast milk doesn't stain baby clothes the way formula does" and "even the baby's poop smells different." Ask around, and mothers will tell you their very own reason to breastfeed.

2. Is breastfeeding that much better than formula?

Yes, because human milk is especially suited to human babies. Milk is species specific. That means that each species of mammal makes milk especially suited to the young of that species. Elephants make elephant milk. Cats make cat milk. Whales make whale milk. Humans make human milk.

Carbohydrates
the chemical name for sugars, starches, and cellulose

The proportion of calories, fat, protein, **carbohydrates**, water, and minerals is unique to each type of mammal. Not surprisingly, mammal babies who need to walk soon after birth—such as horses, goats, and cows—get milk from their mothers that is high in the minerals needed to grow strong bones. Whales make milk that is very high in fat because whale babies need to put on a thick layer of blubber before migrating to colder waters.

What do human babies need? They are helpless compared to other mammals and remain helpless for a long time—it will be months before human babies can walk, so they need to be held and carried around.

Newborn
a human baby younger than 1 month of age

Human **newborns** can focus only on objects about 8–12 inches away—about the distance from the breast to mother's face. So being held at the breast helps with visual development. Unlike mammal babies who develop the ability to stand up and walk early, such as horses, human babies need to develop their brain early—the composition of human milk is perfect for this!

Immunoglobulins
proteins that provide immunity

In addition, milk contains human-specific bioactive components, such as **immunoglobulins**, that provide protection from harmful organisms in the environment.

Over the years the companies that manufacture formula have tried to make formula more and more like breast milk by adding extra ingredients, but every year new components of human milk are discovered and new functions of human milk are found. The species-specific ingredients of your milk can never be duplicated in a laboratory or factory.

In spite of formula's drawbacks, babies who are not fed human milk should be fed manufactured formula for the 1st year—not homemade concoctions, cow's milk, goat's milk, or soy or rice "milks." Never feed your baby anything that your baby's doctor has not approved.

Never feed your baby anything that your baby's doctor has not approved.

Doesn't breastfeeding and all that holding spoil babies?

No! Babies can't be spoiled by having their needs met. While they were in the womb, every need was met. The temperature was perfect and warm, nourishment was constant, and the sound of mother's heartbeat could always be heard. By being held and breastfed when hungry, your baby will be warm, hear your heartbeat, and receive the ideal nourishment. Your baby will learn to trust you, learn that you are loving and welcoming, and learn that needs—like hunger, cold, and loneliness—will be met promptly. Breastfeeding eases the transition from the womb to the world.

Doesn't breastfeeding tie women down?

Nowadays breastfeeding is easier than ever for women to fit into their lives. You can express your milk and refrigerate or freeze it, and then someone else can feed it to the baby when you and the baby are apart. However, there is no doubt that sometimes women feel tied down by motherhood, by having another baby, by the demands of being a mother and a woman today. If they feel as though there is just too much to do, too many demands, too much pressure, they may think that giving up breastfeeding will make their life easier.

Mothers also sometimes worry about how close they feel to their baby. They worry about how important the baby is to them. A mother might worry that she will never be "herself" again. Becoming a mother changes everything—a woman's relationship with her parents, her family, her friends, her job, her daily routine. Breastfeeding underlines these changes by making it very clear, day and night, that she is the mother of the baby.

A woman must make many difficult decisions: Whom should I take care of first? The baby? My partner? My other children? My parents? My friends? My job? Myself? Women may be torn between these conflicting demands. The baby usually doesn't have a voice in the decision, and formula and feeding bottle manufacturers are happy to get another customer.

If you find yourself thinking that if you give up breastfeeding your life would be back to the way it was before you became pregnant, talk over your feelings with someone who has the time to listen and help you think through all your options. Many women have told us that small adjustments in the demands of their lives have made all the difference—getting a more carefree hairdo, preparing simpler meals, making shopping lists, accepting help when it's offered, taking a 20-minute nap, or having a weekly date with their partner or friends.

Won't my partner and my other children feel left out if I breastfeed?

Sometimes other people, both adults and children, feel that the close relationship between the mother and the baby is an exclusive one, that there is no place for them. But babies enjoy time with other people, watching a toddler play, and being skin to skin with another adult. (See Figure 1.) Learning that Dad has a different sound, smell, and feel than Mom helps the baby know that the world has many different qualities. That's an important lesson.

Here are some tips from mothers to help when other children feel left out:

• Use a sling or infant carrier sometimes so that your hands are free to read books or play with your other children.

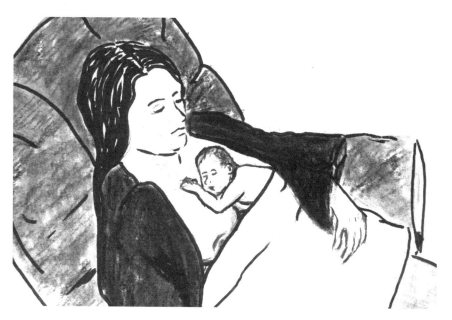

Figure 1 Skin-to-Skin Holding
Skin-to-skin holding warms and comforts babies.

- Keep a box of toys, DVDs, and books that come out only when you're breastfeeding. This will give the other children a treat during nursing times.
- Plan special times for age-appropriate activities for the older children. You can keep the baby close to you in a sling or infant carrier and go for walks, play in the playground, do puzzles, or play games.

Here are some tips from mothers to help when partners feel left out:

- Be careful about criticizing your partner's interactions with the baby. Mothers can fuel feelings of resentment by pointing out "wrong" diapering, clothes put on backward, etc.
- Suggest activities besides diaper changing as ways for your partner to interact with the baby. **Skin-to-skin holding**, bath time, and baby games (like "stick out your tongue and I'll stick out mine") are wonderful ways for adults to interact with a young baby.
- Find special times for the two of you. Even jobs as ordinary as cleaning up the kitchen together can be a time of sharing, a time to talk about your day, a time for a nightly date in the kitchen with the TV off!

James told us, "The baby's mother and I really didn't know each other very well before the baby came. It was really hard for me to see how much attention the baby got. I think I felt really left out and worried if we had what it takes to make a relationship work in the long run. I wondered if the baby would ever love me.

"I didn't have much experience with babies to begin with, and my baby's mother criticized everything I tried to do. Then I found out about skin-to-skin holding. The baby would lie on my chest and snuggle right down. I could watch TV with her right on my chest! I did it every day when I came home from work. When she was a couple of

Skin-to-skin holding

the practice of holding the infant so that his bare chest is against that of his mother or father (the baby is held under the parent's clothing and covered as needed for warmth); this technique helps the baby regulate heart rate, respiratory rate, and body temperature and facilitates early breastfeeding *months old, she started to get excited the minute I put my key in the lock. She holds out her arms to me. It's our special time. I really feel like a dad."*

3. I've heard that breastfeeding is hard to get started. Is it?

Breastfeeding is instinctive for babies, but for mothers, it's a learned skill. In the first hours and days after birth, you and your baby can learn to breastfeed together.

One reason breastfeeding may seem hard is that most of us don't grow up with opportunities to learn how to breastfeed. We bottle-fed our dolls; we grew up seeing women bottle-feeding their babies in public places. We don't tend to see many women breastfeeding in public because breastfeeding can be done so discreetly. Another reason that breastfeeding may seem as if it's hard to do is that you can't practice before your baby is born so you don't know firsthand what it will be like.

It helps to learn more about breastfeeding when you are pregnant. Find answers to your questions. Try to imagine what breastfeeding will be like for you. Where will you sit? Whom will you call if you have questions? Is there a nursing mothers or La Leche group that you could attend during your pregnancy? Is there a peer counselor or mother-to-mother support group leader whom you could call? Could you spend time with a friend or relative who is currently breastfeeding a young baby?

Another way to get ready for breastfeeding is to get ready for your baby's birth:

- Take childbirth classes.
- Take a tour of the hospital or birth center where you will deliver.

Breastfeeding is instinctive for babies, but for mothers, it's a learned skill.

Choosing Breastfeeding

- Go to a prenatal breastfeeding class. Go to a La Leche Meeting or a nursing mother's group meeting.
- If you are a Women, Infants, and Children (WIC) participant, ask for a peer counselor.
- Take a parenting class to learn how to give your baby a bath, take your baby's temperature, etc.
- Find out about doula services. (A doula is trained to mother-the-mother during labor. At-home doula services may also be available in your community to mother-the-mother in her home after the baby is born.)
- Try drug-free ways to minimize the discomfort of labor. Whirlpool baths, birthing balls, massage, hypnosis, and guided imagery are popular techniques you can learn more about.
- Ask that your baby not be given formula without your consent.
- Ask that your baby not be given a pacifier except during painful procedures.
- Ask your visitors to wait until after you are home to see the baby.
- Ask to keep your baby skin-to-skin until after the first self-attached breastfeeding.
- Ask to keep the baby in your room all the time unless there is a medical reason for separation.
- Ask about breastfeeding help in the community. What are the services? Classes? Groups? Consultations? How much do they cost? Who is eligible?

Women have been breastfeeding babies since the dawn of time! Breastfeeding seems hard when you hear all the rules that people like to give you—what you can and cannot eat, what you can and cannot drink, what you can and cannot do. We hope that by reading the questions and answers in this book, you will learn how many of those dos and don'ts are actually old wives' tales.

4. Should every woman breastfeed?

No. The Centers for Disease Control and Prevention's (CDC) list of women who absolutely should not breastfeed is published on its Web site and is revised as information changes. Table 1 lists the reasons that were current at the date of this book's publication. There may be other situations where mothers have had to temporarily stop breastfeeding, but as noted in Table 1, these happen very infrequently.

What about women who have had breast surgery?

Many women who have had cosmetic breast surgery (implants or breast reduction) have gone on to have successful breastfeeding experiences, but it's hard for them to know whether they are making and transferring enough milk to the baby without closely following the baby's weight gain. The concerns are mainly about whether a past surgery has affected the nerves and/or milk-making tissue in the breasts. You cannot really

Table 1   The CDC's List of Women Who Should Not Breastfeed

At the time of publication of this book, the Centers for Disease Control and Prevention advised women not to breastfeed if they:

- Have been infected with the human immunodeficiency virus (HIV)
- Are taking antiretroviral medications
- Have untreated, active tuberculosis
- Are infected with human T-cell lymphotropic virus (HTLV) type 1 or type 2
- Are using or are dependent on an illicit drug
- Are taking prescribed cancer chemotherapy agents, such as antimetabolites, that interfere with DNA replication and cell division
- Are undergoing radiation therapies (such nuclear medicine therapies require only a temporary interruption in breastfeeding)

Source: Adapted from Centers for Disease Control and Prevention. (2007). *When should a mother avoid breastfeeding?* Retrieved September 21, 2007, from http://cdc.gov/breastfeeding/disease/contraindicators.htm

answer these questions until after your baby has been born and you are breastfeeding. Why? Because pregnancy hormones will encourage the growth of your milk-making system and improve your chances of making and delivering an adequate milk supply for the baby. See Question 87 for information about breastfeeding after breast surgery or trauma.

If you've had any breast surgery (cosmetic or otherwise), please be sure that the baby's healthcare provider knows so that your baby can be scheduled for extra weight checks. Plan on having these weight checks until you know that you're making and transferring enough milk, usually for at least the 1st month.

If you've had implants (augmentation), it's especially important not to put too much pressure against your breasts because the implant takes up some of the space inside the breast and puts pressure on the milk-making cells. Pressure on the cells tells them to make less milk. So don't wear a bra that is too tight, and keep your breasts soft by breastfeeding frequently.

If you've had your nipples pierced, you can breastfeed. Take your jewelry out before breastfeeding. If you leak milk though your piercing, use absorbent pads. You can buy them in cloth or paper.

5. Which type of breasts and nipples are not good for breastfeeding?

You can't tell by looking! Breastfeeding relies on the way the breast and nipple function, not the way they look. Women have breastfed with every type of breast and nipple; but **inverted nipples** ("innies") that never come out are probably the most challenging, and many moth-

Inverted nipple

a nipple that turns inward when stimulated

ers with nipples that never protrude find that they have to pump their breasts to maintain their milk supply.

If you have inverted nipples, they may change during pregnancy. After the baby is born, gentle pumping helps many formerly inverted nipples come out. For breastfeeding to be successful, the nipple and breast have to fill the baby's mouth, and that can only happen if the nipple comes out and stretches. Ask yourself, "Is the nipple out in the baby's mouth during the breast-feeding?" Check the second the baby lets go. Do you see the nipple protruding? Can someone else see it? Have a full breastfeeding assessment by a breastfeeding care provider, as well as frequent weight checks in the early days and weeks, to ensure that the baby is gaining weight well.

Women with big breasts or small breasts can make lots of milk: size *doesn't* matter. Rarely, women don't have enough milk-making tissue in their breasts. This ana-tomical problem happened while they were developing as babies inside their mothers. This phenomenon can affect one or both breasts.

Please bring any of the following to the attention of your healthcare or breastfeeding care provider:

- If one breast is considerably smaller or a markedly different shape than the other
- If you do not undergo the expected changes during pregnancy, including:
  - Developing larger breasts
  - Developing a more visible vein pattern under the skin of your breasts

Breastfeeding relies on the way the breast and nipple function, not the way they look.

- A darkening of the skin around your nipples (the **areola**)
- An increase in the size and prominence of the **Montgomery glands** on your areola (Montgomery glands look like goose bumps on the surface of the skin)

Areola

the darkened area around the nipple

Montgomery glands

the small glands of the darker skin of the breast around the nipple. The Montgomery glands become more noticeable during pregnancy. They produce a sticky, shiny antimicrobial lubricant that coats the breast and nipple

Please also report the following experiences to your healthcare provider:

- Any breast surgery, including cosmetic improvements and biopsies
- Any past breast and chest injuries
- If one or both of your nipples don't protrude
- Areas of your breast that have lumps, swelling, redness, or pain
- Anything that concerns you

6. Can every baby breastfeed?

Galactosemia

a rare congenital inability of the body to metabolize the simple sugar galactose, causing damage to the liver, central nervous system, and other body systems

Congenital

a condition that has existed from birth

Central nervous system

the brain and the spinal cord

No. There is one condition that would absolutely not allow breastfeeding—if the baby were diagnosed with **galactosemia**. Galactosemia is a rare **congenital** inability of the body to metabolize the simple sugar, galactose, causing damage to the liver, **central nervous system**, and other body systems. Galactosemia is estimated to occur in 1 of every 60,000 births, and because this condition can quickly lead to death, newborn blood tests screen for it. In the rare situation that a baby is found to be positive for galactosemia, a special prescription formula is required.

There are some infant conditions that can make breastfeeding especially challenging. The most common are covered in Part 7.

7. How long do I have to breastfeed for my baby to get all the immunities?

As long as you breastfeed, your breast milk will continue to have immunities and other protective components. Whenever a breastfeeding mother is exposed to potentially harmful organisms, her immune system creates specific defenders against them and transfers these defenders to her milk. These protective components are listed in Table 2.

In addition, an **exclusively breastfed** baby is not exposed to **contaminants** (e.g., bottles, bottle nipples or teats, water) and not exposed to formula ingredients the way a formula-fed baby is.

Exclusive breastfeeding

when a baby is given no drinks or foods other than breast milk and no pacifiers or artificial nipples

Contaminants

factors that make a product unclean or impure

Table 2   The Protective Components of Human Milk

In addition to having access to the mother's immune system, babies receive the following through breast milk:

- Bifidus factor that promotes the intestinal presence of lactobacillus bifidus, which crowds out pathogenic organisms
- Hormones and hormonelike factors and growth factors that stimulate growth and development of the gastrointestinal (GI) tract and GI motility, such as GI hormones, prolactin, epidermal growth factor, and prostaglandins
- Antibodies, such as SIgA, that bind to microbes in the baby's intestinal tract and prevent them from being absorbed into the rest of the baby's body
- White blood cells—such as B and T lymphocytes, macrophages, and neutrophils—that kill microbes directly or mobilize other defenses
- Cell wall disrupters that kill microbes by destroying the cell wall, including fatty acids and lysozymes
- B_{12} binding factor that reduces the amount of B_{12} in the intestines available to microbes
- Lactoferrin, which has immunoprotective as well as possibly other properties
- Antimicrobial-activity boosters, such as fibronectin and gamma interferon
- Mucosal wall protectors, such as mucins and oligosaccharides, that adhere to microbes and bind them so that they can't attach to the gut wall

Professional and governmental authorities in the United States recommend exclusively breastfeeding (i.e., no other liquids, such as formula or solid foods) for about the first 6 months. Then you should add appropriate **complementary foods** to your baby's diet while continuing to breastfeed through the 1st year—or longer. International authorities, the World Health Organization (WHO), and the United Nations Children's Fund (UNICEF) recommend that breastfeeding should continue for 2 to 3 years.

Complementary food

food other than breast milk that complements, but does not replace, breastfeeding

8. Will breastfeeding "ruin" my breasts?

No, although both men and women have worried about this. Researchers in Italy have recently studied women's breast changes and published their results in a medical journal. Breastfeeding mothers and formula-feeding mothers were asked about their breast changes during pregnancy and after. The conclusion? Some mothers in both groups felt negatively about their breasts. The researchers concluded that changes are more likely to be related to pregnancy, not to breastfeeding.

Will I need to wear a bra day and night if I breastfeed?

No, you don't have to wear a bra, but you might decide to wear one if it makes you feel more comfortable—just be sure that it's not too tight. Pressure on your milk-making cells may send them the message to make less milk if the bra causes less room to store the milk that's already been made.

Nursing bras provide both support and comfort. Some mothers like to wear a soft tank top with a built-in shelf bra. Mothers have told us that they think it's a mistake to buy several of one type of bra until you have given yourself a chance to wash and wear that style. You may need to have bras in different sizes because your breasts will change sizes several times during your nursing experience. For example, your breasts will probably be larger from days 3 to 12 than they will be before or after.

9. Will breastfeeding help me get back to my prepregnancy weight faster?

It depends. Women who exclusively breastfeed (give only breastmilk) for the first 6 months lose more weight than women who both breastfeed and use formula to feed their babies. Women who exclusively formula-feed are the slowest at losing weight.

Another consideration is getting your shape back. In research studies women who breastfeed lose significantly more inches around their belly during the 1st month compared to women who formula-feed their baby. Why? Because the hormone that delivers milk (**oxytocin**) also contracts the uterus and makes it smaller and firmer. By 6 months the difference continued to be noticeable.

Oxytocin
the hormone that makes the milk flow in response to nipple stretching and the newborn baby's hands touching the breast. Oxytocin also contracts the uterus in labor and is released during orgasm

Research has also focused on whether the nursing pattern affects weight loss. Findings indicated that a pattern of more frequent breastfeedings resulted in greater weight loss compared to a pattern of less frequent feedings. In other words, nursing 10–12 times a day would result in more weight loss than nursing 6–8 times a day. That's because the hormone that makes milk also tells the mother's body to move fat to the breast from body storage areas (such as the belly, thighs, and buttocks.) This hormone, prolactin, stays higher with more frequent breast stimulation. The frequent nursing pattern of 10–12 times a day is best for babies too because their stomachs are so small and breast milk is so easy to digest. If you're interested in dieting or exercising while breastfeeding, see Questions 54 and 56.

10. Do I have to change my diet if I'm going to breastfeed?

No. Women all over the world, on very different diets, make milk with only minor variations. Human milk is human milk. You can't alter the major components, such as fat or protein, by changing your diet. You can't make your milk more or less watery by drinking more or less liquids.

But there is a good reason to eat a balanced and nutritious diet—you'll feel better, and you'll find it easier to cope with life.

Most authorities also recommend that you take a multivitamin. This will help your body replenish the nutrients you gave to the baby during pregnancy. You should do this whether or not you breastfeed. Some women— for example, those who follow a vegan diet or who have had gastric bypass surgery—may not have sufficient vitamin B_{12} for themselves or for their breastfed baby. They should discuss their need for vitamin B_{12} with their healthcare provider or with a dietician.

Another special circumstance is for women who live in parts of the world where the diet does not contain recommended amounts of vitamin A and foods are not supplemented with vitamin A. In this case mothers are given vitamin A supplements soon after giving birth.

Breastfeeding decreases a woman's blood loss in the days after the birth and makes it easier for her body to absorb what it needs from the food she eats. Breastfeeding replenishes the body's stores of vitamins and minerals that were transferred to the baby during pregnancy. Women who breastfeed have greater bone mineral density compared to women who don't.

So eat a balanced and nutritious diet for yourself—but not with the mistaken idea that your milk will be of better quality. Please see Question 55 for more information about diet and breastfeeding.

I hate drinking milk. Will I have to drink milk if I choose to breastfeed?

No, you don't have to drink (cow's) milk to make (human) milk.

Will I have to give up my favorite foods, like chocolate?

No, there are no dietary restrictions for breastfeeding mothers, although you may see lists that include onions, chocolate, spicy foods, and so on. There has been some research about foods and breastfeeding. Babies learn to like the foods they taste in the amniotic fluid during pregnancy and in breast milk and then prefer those flavors later when they start eating family foods. This is how we pass on the flavors of our culture. So if you pass up foods that your family eats or that you like to eat, your child could become a picky eater. Research studies indicate that the longer babies are breastfed, the more likely they are to eat family foods and the less likely they are to be problem eaters. For more information about diet and breastfeeding, please see Question 55.

Choosing Breastfeeding

Are there times when pregnant women and breastfeeding mothers have to avoid certain foods?

Yes. Some experts recommend that if there's a history of allergies in the family, the mother should avoid peanuts both while she is pregnant and while she is breastfeeding.

Researchers have found a connection between some colicky breastfed babies and mothers who drink cow's milk. See Question 82 for more on colic.

11. Can I take the same over-the-counter and prescription drugs that I'm taking now in pregnancy when I'm breastfeeding?

It depends on the drug. Because pregnancy and lactation are different physiologic states, drugs that are contraindicated during pregnancy may be acceptable during lactation and vice versa. So it's important to tell all your healthcare providers when you're pregnant or breastfeeding.

Don't think that just because a drug is given by prescription, it's more likely to be a problem for breastfeeding mothers. For both over-the-counter and prescription drugs, the medication, dose, method of administration (e.g., by injection or by mouth), age of the baby, or length of time the mother will take the drug may determine whether the drug is appropriate for use while breastfeeding. Some drugs can affect the baby's behavior. Others can have a negative affect on lactation. For example, pseudoephedrine, a common ingredient in over-the-counter cold and allergy prepa-

Some drugs can affect the baby's behavior. Others can have a negative affect on lactation.

rations, may decrease milk volume. If you need to take a prescription or over-the-counter drug that isn't recommended for breastfeeding mothers, ask your healthcare provider whether there is a safer but equally effective drug that may be substituted.

How about herbs?

Herbs have pharmaceutical properties and can have profound effects on the body, including thinning the blood (i.e., prolonging the time it takes to clot), damaging the liver, raising and lowering the heart rate, and so on. For these and many other reasons, everyone—not just pregnant and nursing mothers—should consider taking herbs with as much or more care than they would manufactured drugs. Many herbal preparations are not manufactured according to pharmaceutical standards. You should always tell your healthcare provider if you're taking any herbal preparations.

12. Can I use recreational drugs, smoke, or drink alcohol while I'm breastfeeding?

No. Recreational (street) drugs are always dangerous to the person taking them, but during pregnancy and lactation, they are dangerous to the baby, too. They are absolutely contraindicated by all health authorities since they are not safe. And there is an additional problem with these drugs—they are illegal. Mothers who have been found to use illegal drugs when pregnant or breastfeeding have been prosecuted, and their babies have been removed from their care.

What about drinking alcohol?

Alcohol in moderation is OK for breastfeeding mothers. According to the Institute of Medicine, alcohol may be consumed by nursing mothers: "If alcohol is used, advise the lactating woman to limit her intake to no more than 0.5 g of alcohol per kg of maternal body weight per day . . . For a 60-kg (132-lb) woman, 0.5 g of alcohol per kg of body weight corresponds to approximately 2 to 2.5 oz of liquor, 8 oz of table wine, or 2 cans of beer.[2]

If I do drink alcohol, should I pump my breasts and discard the milk to get rid of the alcohol in my milk?

No, that is not necessary. Because alcohol is water soluble, it can move from your bloodstream into your milk and then back into your blood. So, by the time you have cleared the alcohol out of your body and you are no longer feeling the effects, it's out of your milk.

What about smoking?

The biggest problem with smoking and babies is secondhand smoke. All babies, no matter how they're fed, should be protected from secondhand smoke. So that's the first priority: protect yourself while you're pregnant, and protect yourself and your baby after the birth. Don't forget to protect your baby from secondhand smoke in cars. If you're out of doors, move your baby away from anyone who is smoking.

Even if you have tried to quit smoking before and failed, try again now. It's worth it. You're worth it.

Smoking isn't contraindicated (nor forbidden) for breastfeeding mothers, but if you do smoke, it's best for your own health to quit. There are many proven ways to help people stop smoking. Talk to your healthcare provider about what techniques could work for you.

[2]Institute of Medicine. (1991) *Nutrition during lactation*. Washington, DC: National Academy of Sciences.

Even if you have tried to quit smoking before and failed, try again now. It's worth it. You're worth it.

13. How do I know whether my milk is going to be any good?

Although this is a common question, research indicates that the quality of milk doesn't vary very much from one woman to another.

One reason a woman may become concerned about the quality of her milk is that she is not familiar with the normal appearance of human milk. She may compare her milk to homogenized cow's milk and think that her milk looks thin and bluish. She may believe that it's weak or low in quality.

Human milk's appearance changes over the course of lactation. A woman's body begins to make early milk, **colostrum**, around the middle of pregnancy. It's thick, yellow, and compact—perfect for a newborn baby who is learning how to coordinate **sucking**, swallowing, and breathing. Although a woman begins to make mature milk soon after she delivers the placenta, that milk will continue to have colostral components for a few days. The presence of colostrum makes the milk look thicker and more yellow. After there are no longer colostral components in the milk, it is whiter and bluer.

Around the 3rd day after the baby is born, the volume of milk increases dramatically. Mothers notice that their breasts are firmer and fuller. But the increase in size is not just because of the increase in milk volume. There is also an increase in blood flow and lymphatic activity that makes the breasts larger and firmer. This will subside around the beginning of the 2nd week.

Colostrum

the first milk, produced in the breasts by the 5th month of pregnancy—colostrum is thick, sticky, and clear to yellowish in color; is high in protein and vitamin A; causes a laxative effect, helping the baby pass meconium; and contains immunoglobulins (mostly IgA), which protect the baby from infections

Sucking

drawing into the mouth by forming a partial vacuum with the lips and tongue

Then the breasts will feel softer and be noticeably smaller. This change may coincide with the absence of noticeable colostral components in the milk. A mother could get the mistaken idea that the softer breasts and whiter milk mean that the quantity and or quality of her milk has changed for the worse.

Is breast milk polluted? There was a news story about environmental contaminants in breast milk.

Samples of human milk (along with other samples of the environment such as fish, groundwater, air, snow, and bird's eggs) are examined year after year to detect whether the planet has gotten more or less polluted, what chemicals are found in the samples, and also to estimate the human exposure to the chemical contaminants. Why is human milk on the list? Not because it is more or less polluted but because it is a fatty human tissue that is safe and easy for the researchers to obtain.

Is this something I should be worried about?

No. A baby is most exposed to the pollutants in the mother's body during pregnancy, not during breastfeeding. The only cause for concern is if you have been notified that you were personally exposed through an accidental occupational or environmental event.

If you are concerned about your milk, either the quantity or quality, talk to your healthcare provider, your baby's healthcare provider, or a breastfeeding care provider.

14. Women in my family have had a hard time with breastfeeding, so it probably won't work for me, right?

Being physically unable to breastfeed isn't something that runs in families, but families for whom breastfeeding is unfamiliar may have a lot of unhelpful mistaken ideas about breastfeeding and may not be supportive of a family member's decision to breastfeed. A mother has to learn to breastfeed, and if you haven't had an opportunity to learn as you were growing up, you can learn on the job.

When you are pregnant, you can read, talk to other mothers, spend time with women who are breastfeeding, and line up your sources of breastfeeding information and support. Try to visualize what breastfeeding will be like for you.

Mothers tell us that it was helpful to listen to the stories of other family members who have had negative breastfeeding experiences. It helps women to talk about what happened to them, and hearing their story may help you. After listening, ask these women for support for your breastfeeding journey.

15. Can I get pregnant when I'm breastfeeding?

Yes. Breastfeeding does not keep you from getting pregnant, but for women who aren't trying to prevent future pregnancies, those who breastfeed have longer spaces in between babies. If a woman does get pregnant while she is breastfeeding, she can usually continue to breastfeed while pregnant. She may go on to nurse both babies. This is called **tandem nursing**. For information about nursing during pregnancy and tandem nursing, please see Questions 72–73.

Tandem nursing
nursing two children of different pregnancies—for example, a newborn and a toddler

PART TWO

Getting Started with Breastfeeding

When should I start breastfeeding?

What are the ways I could position myself and the baby for breastfeeding?

What should breastfeeding feel like?

More ...

16. How do the breasts make milk?

The breasts make milk in milk-making cells that are formed during fetal development. All babies, boys and girls, are born with these cells and have the possibility to make milk. Girls' bodies develop the milk-making potential further during puberty, when hormones increase the size of girls' breasts as well as the amount of functional tissue. This is visible as breast buds and later as developed breasts. With each menstrual cycle a woman's breasts, as well as her uterus, prepare for pregnancy and lactation. If there is no pregnancy, the cycle begins again.

When pregnancy does occur, the milk-making cells continue to develop. The breasts enlarge, and the Montgomery glands become more prominent, standing out on the areola and secreting a sticky, antimicrobial lubricant onto the nipple, areola, and breast. Veins in the breast become more obvious, indicating the increased blood flow to the milk-making cells.

Many women also notice that their areola, the darker area of skin around the nipple, darkens further. They produce their first milk, colostrum, around the middle of pregnancy and continue to produce it while pregnancy hormones are present in their body.

The baby's suckling in the first hours and days after birth primes receptor sites on the surface of the milk-making cells to respond to the hormone **prolactin.** This hormone is essential for ongoing milk production. Around the 3rd day after birth, hormone changes result in the production of an abundant amount of mature milk. This change is evident visually as the look of colostrum, thick and yellow, gives way to thin, blue-white mature milk. Colostrum will continue to be

Prolactin

hormone that stimulates milk production

mixed into the mature milk for days to come. Milk that contains both colostrum and mature milk is commonly called "transitional milk" and lasts into the 2nd week.

Milk production requires two main influences—the stimulation of suckling and the absence of pressure on the milk-making cells. The pattern of short frequent nursings, about 10–12 times a day beginning shortly after birth, is optimal for both the ongoing production of milk and the nutrition and nurture of the baby. Why? Because human breast milk is easy to digest and babies thrive on such activities as being held and touched, seeing their mother's face, and being warm— which they get, along with optimal nutrition, when being breastfed.

17. Should I do anything during pregnancy to get my breasts and nipples ready for breastfeeding?

No. Pregnancy hormones will prepare your breasts and nipples for breastfeeding. This happens whether or not you choose to breastfeed. Your body will begin to make colostrum, and your milk will increase in abundance in the early days postpartum. In the past women were advised to prepare their breasts and nipples in a variety of ways, including through exercise, exposure to sunlight, scrubbing, using creams and lotions, and wearing devices inside the bra. Research has shown that none of these suggestions actually helps. If, at the end of pregnancy, one or both of your nipples is inverted, see Question 76.

There is one thing you can do during pregnancy that is helpful—discover where to get breastfeeding help.

18. Where can I get breastfeeding help?

Communities offer women a variety of ways to get individualized breastfeeding assessment, education, and support. You can do a community inventory. Make a list of all the possibilities. Ask about cost and insurance coverage.

Find out the answers to these questions:

- Does your birthing facility have trained staff? Has the facility received the WHO/UNICEF **Baby-Friendly Hospital** designation for implementing the "**Ten Steps to Successful Breastfeeding**"?
- Which pediatric practice do you plan to use? Ask whether staff members follow the recommendations of their national pediatric authority. Where do they recommend that you receive your postpartum breastfeeding assessments? How do they manage questions and routine weight checks? If you want to know your baby's weight, will the nurse weigh your baby during office hours? Is there a breastfeeding care provider on staff? If not, how does the office handle breastfeeding questions and problems?
- Is there a peer counselor program available for you beginning in pregnancy? How does the peer counselor program function? Are there group meetings that you can begin attending while pregnant?
- Are there **doulas** in your community? What services do they offer? Do they give childbirth as well as postpartum support?
- Do visiting nurses or health visitors make home visits to new mothers in your community? Does your insurance pay for these visits? In some communities every new mother is entitled to one public health nursing visit and more if there are any concerns.

Communities offer women a variety of ways to get individualized breastfeeding assessment, education, and support.

Baby-Friendly Hospital Initiative (BFHI)

a United Nations Children's Fund and World Health Organization program recognizing hospitals and birth centers that implement the "Ten Steps to Successful Breastfeeding"

"Ten Steps to Successful Breastfeeding"

guidelines developed by the United Nations Children's Fund (UNICEF) and the World Health Organization (WHO) that protect and promote breastfeeding in facilities that provide maternity services and care for newborn infants—see **Baby-Friendly Hospital Initiative**

Doula

an individual who supports the mother during the perinatal period, colloquially known as "mothering the mother"

33

- Is there a La Leche group or nursing mothers group nearby? Are there baby cafés or "nursing nooks" where you can drop in? What programs are available?
- Are breastfeeding care providers available in your community? Does the provider have a certificate of added knowledge? The Academy of Breastfeeding Medicine, the Academy of Lactation Policy and Practice, and the International Board of Lactation Consultant Examiners are among the agencies that provide credentials in lactation management. What is the person's background in addition to lactation credentials? Find out about the services the breastfeeding care provider offers.
- Is there a warmline or hotline for breastfeeding mothers in your area? A live person usually answers a warmline during some hours, and questions or issues left on the warmline's answering machine are responded to promptly with a return call. A hotline is always answered live. Give these resources a call.
- Are the telephone numbers you've been given working? Call to make sure.

Breastfeeding works best if you start as soon as possible after you give birth and then nurse frequently.

Hypoglycemia

low blood sugar

Jaundice

a condition that results when red blood cells break down faster than the liver can handle, yellowing the skin; in the newborn, normal physiologic jaundice is caused by the immaturity of the liver

Hyperbilirubinemia

high levels of bilirubin in the blood

After you have compiled a list of breastfeeding helpers in your community, ask mothers about the help and support they received. Did these resources meet the mothers' breastfeeding goals? If they had problems with breastfeeding, were those problems solved? Were these mothers treated the way you would like to be treated?

19. When should I start breastfeeding?

Breastfeeding works best if you start as soon as possible after you give birth and then nurse frequently. Common problems with newborns, such as low blood sugar (**hypoglycemia**) and **jaundice** (**hyperbilirubinemia**), may be prevented or lessened in severity when babies are breastfed soon after birth and then frequently in the first days. Breastfeeding works best if you nurse 30–35 times in the first 3 days. You will want to keep your baby near you so that you can nurse whenever you see feeding cues. (See Figures 2–5.) If you use the self-attached and collaborative breastfeeding techniques described in Question 20, breastfeeding will be easy and fun.

20. How do I start breastfeeding?

Normal breastfeeding progresses through two phases. In the first phase the baby self-attaches to the breast using the stepping-crawling reflex; this is *self-attached breastfeeding*. In the second phase the mother and baby work together to achieve the latch and feeding; this is *collaborative breastfeeding*.

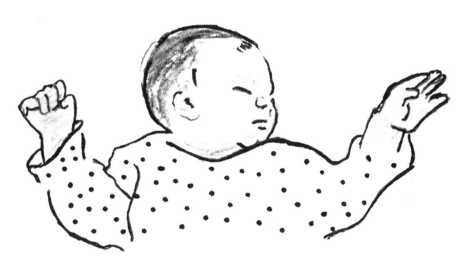

Figure 2 Feeding Cues (a)
Subtle body motions are a feeding cue.

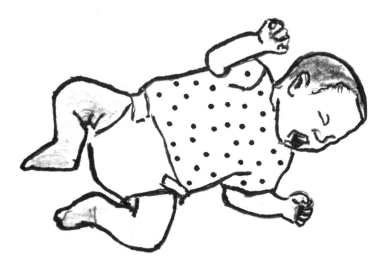

Figure 3 Feeding Cues (b)
Mouthing is a feeding cue (the baby may make little sucking noises).

Start by holding your baby skin to skin, and move to self-attached breastfeeding, where your baby takes the lead. In the first days try more and more collaborative breastfeeding, where you and the baby work together. Self-attached breastfeeding uses the baby's innate skill and ability to locate the nipple and begin breastfeeding. Collaborative breastfeeding is more of what people imagine breastfeeding to be—the mother and baby work to achieve breastfeeding together.

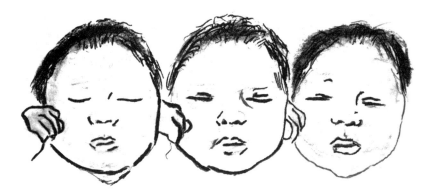

Figure 4 Feeding Cues (c)
Rapid eye movement is a feeding cue.

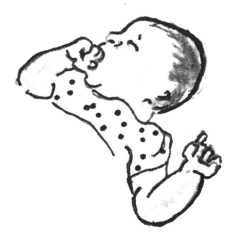

Figure 5 Feeding Cues (d)
Putting the hand near the mouth is a feeding cue.

Self-Attached Breastfeeding

Self-attached breastfeeding should begin as soon as possible after birth. It begins with skin-to-skin holding and allows the baby to use a stepping-crawling motion to approach the breast, nuzzle, and nurse. This journey may take more than 2 hours if the mother received drugs in labor, less if she did not. If the birth was by cesarean, skin-to-skin holding and self-attached breastfeeding can begin as soon as the mother has recovered enough to respond to the baby—in the delivery room, in the recovery area, or in her hospital room. Until the mother is ready, the father or another adult can hold the baby skin to skin.

To begin skin-to-skin holding, the healthy baby is dried and put on the mother's chest. Both mother and baby are then covered with a warmed blanket, and a little soft cap is put on the baby's head. The baby is usually positioned between the mother's breasts. The baby goes through stages of awakening and approaches the breast using a stepping-crawling motion. The baby will

37

find the nipple, nuzzle, and ideally, begin to nurse. This is an opportunity for the mother's body to warm the baby. She actually does this better than hospital warming cribs, according to research. The mother's breasts keep the baby at the right temperature.

Collaborative Breastfeeding

With collaborative breastfeeding, as the baby seeks the breast, the mother gently assists. The mother uses her body—her arms, hands, and lap—to hold the baby. Initiate collaborative breastfeeding when you feel ready.

First, observe that your baby is showing feeding cues, described in Table 3.

Crying is considered a late feeding cue because intact full-term babies do not usually cry until more subtle cues have failed to get the mother's attention. Less mature and more disorganized babies pass quickly from the state of deep sleep, characterized by no rapid eye movement (REM), to crying. Wash your hands, and start collaborative feeding right after you see a cue. If you stop to change the diaper or anything else that

Table 3   Feeding Cues

Rooting

natural instinct of the newborn to turn his head toward the nipple and open his mouth when mouth area is gently stroked with the nipple

- **Rooting** and turning the head, especially with searching movements of the mouth
- Increasing alertness, especially rapid eye movement (REM) under closed eyelids
- Flexing of the legs and arms
- Bringing a hand to the mouth (the baby does not have to be successful)
- Sucking on a fist or finger
- Mouthing motions of the lips and tongue
- Head bobbing

takes too much time, your baby may sleep or fret at the breast instead of nursing.

When using the collaborative breastfeeding strategy, your body (especially your arms, hands, and torso) provides the frame and the support needed to keep your baby at your breast. You should find a comfortable posture and make your breast accessible to the baby, allowing the baby the freedom required to achieve pain-free suckling with maximal milk transfer. Please see Question 22 for latch-on information.

21. What are the ways I could position myself and the baby for breastfeeding?

With collaborative breastfeeding, after the baby shows the feeding cues described in Table 3, the mother makes herself comfortable and makes her breast accessible. The baby will begin to seek the breast, and then the mother gently helps the baby latch on.

Your body (especially your arms, hands, and torso) provides the frame or support in collaborative breastfeeding. A variety of common body positions are described next. You should find the postures that are comfortable and allow your baby the freedom to suckle and transfer the maximum amount of milk. You should feel gentle tugging, not pain, if the latch is correct.

Sitting postures include the cradle (Madonna), the cross-cradle, and the clutch (football). In the **cradle** or **Madonna posture** (see Figure 6), the baby lies on his side, facing the mother, with the side of his head and body resting on the forearm of the mother next to the breast to be used.

Cradle or Madonna posture

a breastfeeding posture in which the mother holds the baby on her lap with his head resting on her forearm directly in front of the breast

Getting Started with Breastfeeding

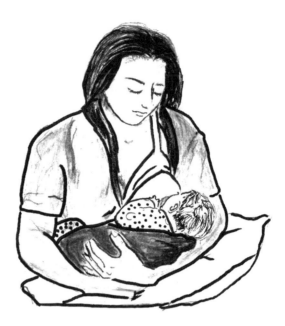

Figure 6 The Cradle Posture
In the cradle posture, the mother supports the baby with the same arm as the breast that the baby is nursing from (also called the Madonna posture).

Cross-cradle posture

a breastfeeding posture in which the mother holds the baby on her lap with his head resting on her forearm of the arm opposite the suckled breast; the hand of her arm on the same side either supports the breast or is free

Football or clutch posture

a breastfeeding posture in which the baby is tucked under the mother's arm, with baby's feet behind his mother's back and the baby's shoulders supported in the palm of her hand

With the **cross-cradle posture** (see Figure 7), the baby lies on his side, facing the mother, with his side resting on the forearm of the mother on the opposite side of the breast being used. This posture is considered especially useful for the mother of a newborn or preterm baby.

The **football** or **clutch posture** (see Figure 8) is another sitting position, in which the baby lies on his side or back, curled between the side of the mother's chest and her arm. The baby's upper body is supported by the mother's forearm. The mother's hand supports the baby's neck and shoulders. The baby's hips are flexed up along a chair back or other surface that the mother is leaning against.

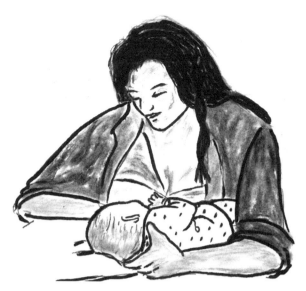

Figure 7 The Cross-Cradle Posture
Using the cross-cradle posture, the mother holds the baby with the arm oppo-site the breast (note that the mother's hand is not putting pressure on the back of the baby's head).

You may also lie back or recline to breastfeed. Many mothers enjoy nursing in a semireclining posture. You lean back, and the baby lies against your body, chest to chest. (See Figure 9.)

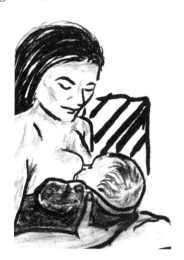

Figure 8 The Football or Clutch Posture
In the football posture, the baby's legs extend under the mother's arm.

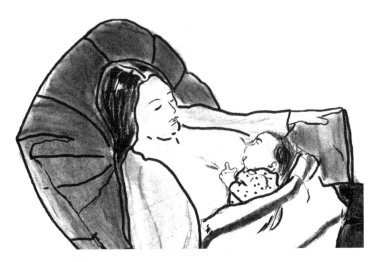

Figure 9   Semireclining Posture
In the semireclining posture, the mother's body supports the baby (note that the baby's head and body are free to move).

To nurse lying down, lie on your side (using the side-lying posture) or on your back (in the Australian posture). When using the side-lying posture, lie on your side. Put the baby chest to chest with you. (See Figure 10.) In the Australian posture you're "down under," lying on your back, with the baby supported on your chest. (See Figure 11.)

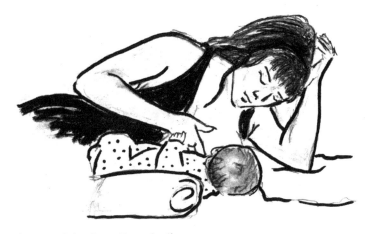

Figure 10   Lying-Down Breastfeeding
Mothers can nurse lying down.

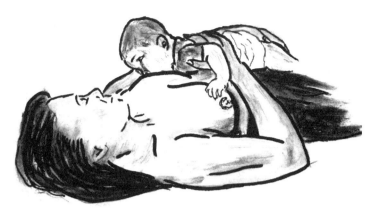

Figure 11 The Australian Posture
When using the Australian posture, the mother is "down under."

22. How should the baby latch onto the breast?

When you're in a comfortable posture and the baby is positioned near your breast, use your hand to support the baby's shoulder at the base of the neck. Be careful not to apply pressure against the back of the baby's head with your arm, your hand, or a pillow. (See Figure 12.) Why? Because the baby's head must be able to tilt back during the latching-on process. Move the baby toward your breast—not the breast to the baby. Don't change the shape of the breast with your hand, and don't push your nipple into the baby's mouth.

Move the baby toward your breast— not the breast to the baby.

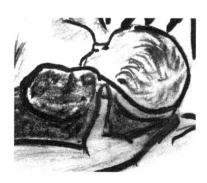

Figure 12 Hand Position
It's important that there's no pressure on the back of the baby's head.

43

Collaborative Latch-On: Step-by-Step

1. Get comfortable in the posture of your choice, and put the baby close to your breast in the position of your choice. Free your breast. Make sure your bra is not pressing anywhere on your breast.

2. There is usually no need to hold your breast while nursing. If you wish to support your breast, it's best to do so in a way that keeps your fingers away from the nipple and does not put pressure on the **milk ducts**. A good way to do this is by putting your hand flat against your chest, under your breast, with your thumb up and over your breast. Make your hand come up as high as possible into the crease. This will bring your breast out away from your chest. You could also roll a facecloth or small towel and put it under your breast as high as possible.

3. Use your hand to cup the baby's shoulders and the base of the baby's neck (not the back of his head).

4. The baby's arms shouldn't cross in front of his body or be swaddled. Let his arms be out and go up around the breast, almost like a hug.

5. The baby should be tummy to tummy with you.

6. Start with the baby's nose opposite your nipple. (See Figure 13.)

7. Bring the baby back away from the breast (about 1–3 inches).

8. As the baby's mouth opens wide (gapes), his head will tilt back slightly during the latch. (See Figure 14.)

9. Move the baby to the breast. Do not direct the breast to the baby. In the football or the cross-cradle hold, place your hand on the base of the baby's neck, and bring him to you. If you're holding the baby in a cradle hold, place the baby's head on your forearm, not in the crook of your elbow,

Milk duct

the narrow tube structure that carries milk to the nipple

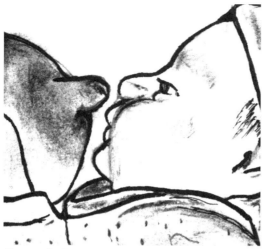

Figure 13 Nose to Nipple
Start with the baby's nose opposite your nipple.

and bring your arm in to move the baby to the breast. The nipple has to be positioned between the tongue and the roof of the baby's mouth, so bringing him to the nipple works best.

10. The baby's tongue extends over his lower lip, and his chin reaches the breast first. The baby's

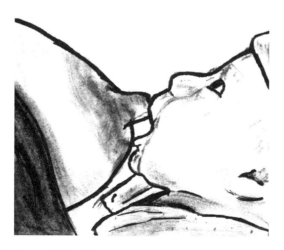

Figure 14 Gape and Head Tilt
The baby's head tilts back, and the mouth gapes. The lower lip and chin reach the breast first.

mouth is wide open as it reaches the breast. (See Figure 15.)

11. The latch should be asymmetric. More of the top of the areola will be showing and less of the bottom of the areola will be visible. (See Figure 16.)

12. The lips should make a seal around the breast. They may look flanged, sort of like a fish.

13. The baby's nose should be close to the breast. His chin may be closer.

14. The corner of the baby's mouth will make an angle greater than 140°.

15. The cheeks will look full, not dimpled or drawn in.

16. The baby begins to suck and swallow. The jaw motion should extend back to the baby's ear. (See Figure 17.) After the first few days, you will hear the baby swallow.

17. When milk is flowing you can see a "rocker-like" motion of the baby's jaw. The baby swings the jaw forward from the area near the ear, using the cheek muscles to move the jaw toward the breast, and

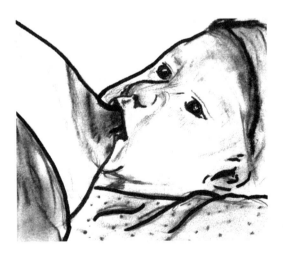

Figure 15 Nipple in Top Half
The tongue takes up half of the mouth. The nipple should be positioned in the top half of the mouth.

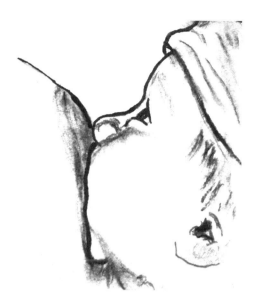

Figure 16 Asymmetric Latch
The baby is positioned asymmetrically at the breast.

then drawing it back. If you see mostly "up and down" motion of the baby's lips, the baby may not be well latched. Consider breaking suction and starting over. To break suction, insert your clean finger in the corner of the baby's mouth, or squash

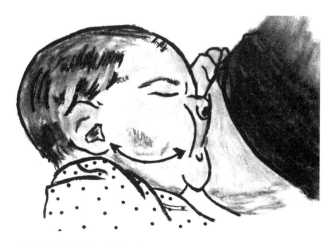

Figure 17 Rocker Motion of the Jaw
The rocker motion of the jaw is associated with the transfer of milk.

your breast toward the far side of the baby's mouth, until the baby releases the breast. Don't just pull the baby off the breast—that hurts!

Breastfeeding should not hurt if the baby is latched correctly. At the most, you might feel a gentle tugging. At the end of the feeding, your nipple should be shaped as it was before the baby latched on.

23. Why should I bother with breastfeeding in the first few days if I haven't made any milk yet?

You will have milk from the minute your baby is born.

You will have milk from the minute your baby is born. Early milk, colostrum, is even available for prematurely born babies. Colostrum is especially suited to the newly born baby because it's packed with immune properties, fat, and protein. Colostrum doesn't spray because it's so densely packed. While getting colostrum, the baby can learn to coordinate sucking, swallowing, and breathing without having to cope with the consistency of mature milk or manufactured infant formula.

Human babies are born without the important immunoglobulin, IgA, which coats all the mucous membranes of adults and protects from organisms in the environment. Colostrum is full of IgA and from the baby's first nursing begins to protect your baby.

While you're breastfeeding and giving your baby colostrum, your milk-making cells and hormones get the message to produce milk.

24. What if my baby doesn't want to breastfeed?

Hold your baby skin to skin. Babies respond to their mother's smell and heartbeat. Babies feed best when nursed at *their* best time. If the baby does not seem to be demanding to breastfeed, watch carefully for feeding cues. Babies normally cycle into rapid eye movement (REM) sleep every half hour or so. REM and quiet alert states are ideal for starting to breastfeed. In the "quiet alert" state the baby is very still but the eyes are wide open and focused, often on a face or round object 8 to 12 inches away—the distance babies see best. Because the baby is concentrating very hard in this state it's ideal for learning how to latch-on and transfer milk from the breast.

Once you see a feeding cue, move to feed the baby right away. Get an individualized breastfeeding assessment from a skilled breastfeeding caregiver if the baby continues to be disinterested in feeding. Get medical help if the baby has fewer stools or wet diapers or has any other of the behaviors listed in Table 4.

What if my baby is hard to wake to feed?

It may be that you're missing feeding cues or feeding at a time that is not the best for the baby. Some babies (e.g., those with **Down syndrome**) are a challenge to feed because their cues are subtle. See Question 95 for more information about breastfeeding and Down syndrome.

One concern about babies who are difficult to wake to feed is that this can be a sign of **malnutrition** or **dehydration**. Other signs are fewer bowel movements and

Down syndrome

a congenital condition characterized by moderate to severe mental retardation, also called "Down's" or "trisomy 21"

Malnutrition

refers to those who are either overfed, underfed, or unable to correctly use the food they're receiving

Dehydration

a condition in which the infant is not receiving adequate fluids or is unable to maintain adequate hydration because of a metabolic reason; symptoms of this potentially serious problem include lethargy (extreme fatigue and weakness), sunken eyes, a sunken soft spot on the infant's head, and little or no urine

Table 4   When to Call for Urgent Medical Help for Your Baby

Consider these questions:

- Is the baby extremely lethargic or irritable?
- Is there a sudden change in the baby's muscle tone (e.g., the baby is extremely stiff or floppy), or is the baby presenting repetitive jerking movements (e.g., seizure activity)?
- Does the baby show a sudden disinterest in feeding?
- Are you unable to wake the baby?
- Does the baby not calm down, even with cuddles?
- Is the baby having meconium (black or tarlike) bowel movements after 5 days of life?
- If the baby is breastfed, does he have fewer than three bowel movements daily after the first 2 days of life?
- Has the baby had no urine in 6 hours?
- If the baby is breastfed, does he have brick dust (red colored) urine daily after 5 days of life?
- Does the baby have noticeably sunken fontanels (soft spots on the top of the baby's head)?
- Is the baby less active?
- Is the baby below his birth weight at 10–14 days of life?
- Has the baby stopped gaining weight?
- Is the baby sleeping at the breast?

If you answered yes to any of those questions, please seek pediatric care now.

decreased urination. If your baby has these symptoms, please seek medical attention immediately.

What if my baby latches but doesn't feed, falls asleep, or doesn't stay attached for the feeding?

If you delay by changing the diaper or doing another activity after the baby has given a feeding cue, the baby is more likely to fret or sleep at the breast. If you have brought the baby to the breast without delay and the baby latches but doesn't suckle, stroke your hand down the breast. This may begin the milk flow, and the baby will swallow. Stroke again, and the baby will swallow.

This is called "alternate massage" or "breast compression" (see Figure 18).

What if my baby won't stop crying?

Babies don't cry only when they are hungry. Check to see whether anything is pinching or hurting the baby. Lots of things can make a baby cry—a hair wrapped tightly around a toe or finger, a skin or diaper rash. Her diaper could have been put on too tightly; her toes could be cramped inside a too small stretch suit. Even when the problem has been taken care of, she may keep crying.

Babies may also cry because they're cold and lonely. Put the baby on your chest, skin to skin. Cover the baby for warmth, leaving her head out. Now she can hear the familiar heartbeat. Your body and breast temperature will warm her up. Usually, a baby will calm when cuddled skin to skin and then move toward the breast.

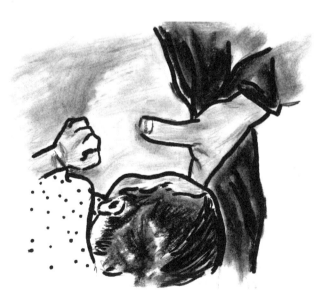

Figure 18   Alternate Massage (Breast Compression)
Alternate compression increases the flow of milk to the baby. The mother compresses the breast when the baby pauses.

If your baby doesn't calm when cuddled or has other symptoms—such as a fever, vomiting, diarrhea, or any other symptom in Table 4—please call for medical help right away.

25. How often do I need to breastfeed?

Breastfeeding works best in a pattern of frequent feedings, 10–12 times a day in the early weeks. Watch the baby, not the clock. Breastfeedings need to be efficient and effective in transferring milk. Babies should nurse until they're finished on one breast. Then the mother should offer the other breast. Some babies will want to nurse right away on the second side; others will need a little nap first. As the early days pass and your milk changes from colostrum to mature milk, you and your baby will develop the pattern that is right for you.

Babies, especially newborns, typically cluster-feed.

Breastfeedings are usually not spaced evenly around the clock. Babies, especially newborns, typically cluster-feed. That is, they have several nursings close together and then space other nursings further apart. At first, many babies' days and nights are mixed up, but if a mother pays attention to feeding cues in the daytime and nurses frequently according to her baby's cues, the nighttime feedings will begin to space out.

How long should a breastfeeding last?

It depends. As a general rule, full-term newborns can efficiently and effectively transfer milk faster than near-term babies. As a group, prematurely born babies transfer milk at the slowest rate. Mothers of prematurely born babies express their breast milk, which is fed to the babies by tube, before they begin breastfeeding. When prematurely born babies or near-term babies are able to breastfeed, each nursing takes longer than it does for full-term babies.

Some babies:

- Nurse from both breasts at each feeding right from the beginning.
- Nurse from just one breast most of the time.
- Take a while to get started with the milk transfer part of nursing. They spend minutes familiarizing themselves with the breast and nipple. Then they latch on and begin nursing in a way that effectively transfers milk. (Be sure you don't put pressure against the back of the baby's head or try to aggressively force the baby to the breast while your baby is latching on and off during familiarization.)
- Latch on and start nursing vigorously and then rest for a few minutes while maintaining a nursing position. Then they nurse vigorously again. The mother can gently massage her breast (called "alternate massage" or "breast compression"; see Question 24), and the baby usually begins to breastfeed vigorously again.

After the early days, efficient and effective full-term babies nurse between 15 and 20 minutes. If your baby is full term, more than 4 days old, and nurses more than 20 minutes or less than 15, ask for an individualized breastfeeding assessment from your breastfeeding caregiver or healthcare provider. This assessment may identify ways to improve the baby's position or latch.

Contrary to popular belief, babies who nurse for longer times often transfer less milk than babies who nurse about 15–20 minutes. Research indicates that babies who ineffectively and inefficiently transfer milk actually give their mother's breasts and hormones the message to make *less* milk over time.

The feeding should end when the baby latches off on her own. Her hands will open and arms will go limp. Her body tone will be soft. (See Figure 19.) If one hand is limp and the other clenched and tight when the baby latches off, she will usually want to nurse again in a little while. (See Figure 20.)

What about getting enough of the highest fat milk, the hindmilk?

Babies need the fat in breast milk for their body functions, brain and nervous system development, and energy. Today, because of excellent research studies, we have a better understanding of fat and breastfeeding.

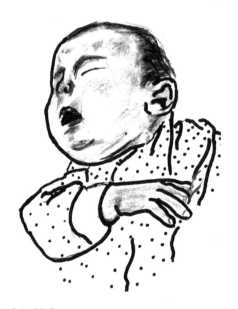

Figure 19 Satiated Baby
When the baby has had enough milk, his hands and body will relax.

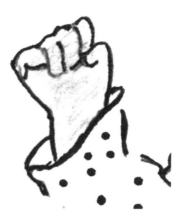

Figure 20 Clenched Fist
If the baby clenches his fist, he will probably want to nurse again.

The Old Idea

In the past people believed that the milk at the end of the nursing, the hind milk, was always higher in fat than the rest of the milk, including the milk at the beginning of the feeding, the **foremilk**. People, therefore, thought that each breastfeeding should last a long time so that the baby would get to the hind milk. If a baby was not gaining enough weight, mothers were told to make the nursing last longer.

The New Idea

Our new understanding, based on well-done research, indicates that babies get ideal amounts of fat with effective and efficient breastfeedings, not according to how long their nursings last.

We now know that sometimes the milk at the end of a nursing is higher in fat, and sometimes it's not. Sometimes the milk at the beginning and the end of the breastfeeding has the same proportion of fat. We know that the proportion of fat and the volume of milk vary

Foremilk

the milk present in the breast at the beginning of a breastfeed by the time of day (there's often more fat in the evening and higher volume in the morning, for example).

Research has also found that the speed of milk removal influences the amount of fat in the milk, so effective, efficient breastfeedings are best.

Wouldn't it be better to put the baby on a schedule right from the beginning?

No. Babies and mothers do best at first with frequent feedings according to the baby's cues. Responding to your baby's needs encourages feelings of security and trust. Babies who have breastfeeding interactions with their mothers are less likely to be picky eaters as toddlers, and their families experience less mealtime conflict.

26. My sister told me that breastfeeding hurts. Should it?

No. Breastfeeding should be a pleasurable experience—the nursing itself, the joy of seeing your baby thrive on your milk, and knowing you're doing the best thing for yourself, your baby, and your family should feel great. Efficient and effective breastfeeding feels like gentle tugging to some women and gentle massage to others.

Women who do not get adequate breastfeeding help may experience pain. Our research shows that, in almost every case, breastfeeding pain in the newborn period is a symptom of poor latch. Individualized assessment and correction of the latch reduces the pain immediately, eliminating it completely within a few feedings.

Breastfeeding pain is a loud and clear message to get help! Follow the tips described in Question 18. If anyone tells you that your pain is normal and to tough it out until it goes away, get help from someone else.

Breastfeeding pain is discussed further in Questions 35, 74, and 75.

27. What happens to breastfeeding plans if the mother or the baby has postpartum complications?

Even if the mother and baby are separated by complications at first, breastfeeding is still possible. If the problem is with the baby, the mother can keep up her milk supply and collect milk for her baby by expressing her milk. She should begin expressing by 6 hours after the birth and express at least eight times a day. If the baby can't go right to the breast because of complications, mother's milk can be fed by tube, by cup, and sometimes by bottle.

If the problem is with the mother, she can maintain the possibility of breastfeeding by expressing her milk. Be sure that everyone knows how important breastfeeding is so that they will make decisions to best preserve lactation. Special situations are described in more detail in Part 7.

28. Should the baby get some formula in the first days when I have only colostrum?

Colostrum is the perfect food for the baby in the first days, providing optimal nutrition along with wonderful immunities. It's best if formula is given to the breastfed baby only for medical reasons. Table 5 lists accepted

Table 5   Acceptable Medical Indications for Giving Formula Supplements to a Breastfed Baby (WHO/UNICEF)

- Infants with severe dysmaturity
- Infants with a very low birth weight
- Infants with inborn errors of metabolism
- Infants with acute water loss
- Infants whose mothers are severely ill
- Infants whose mothers require a medication that is contraindicated

medical reasons, according to the World Health Organization and the United Nations Children's Fund, for supplementing a breastfed infant.

29. What should breastfeeding feel like?

Breastfeeding should always be pleasurable, but the feelings are not the same for every woman. The breastfeeding experience changes as the baby grows and develops and is different from baby to baby. Some of the sensations women experience include:

- Tingling. Some women feel a sensation like ginger ale bubbles in their breast as the milk flows. Many women do not. Don't feel concerned if you don't feel this sensation. You will know that your milk is flowing because, after the first few days, you will hear your baby swallowing. After a small expected weight loss in the early days, your baby will gain about a half ounce to an ounce a day.
- Tugging. A tugging sensation is common as the nipple stretches back into the baby's mouth.
- Pain. Pain is common but not normal. It's a signal to get an individualized breastfeeding assessment.
- Sleepy and relaxed. Some of the hormones that the mother's body releases while she is breastfeeding may make her eyes feel heavy and her body feel

Pain is common but not normal. It's a signal to get an individualized breastfeeding assessment.

lethargic, especially in the early days. These feelings remind the breastfeeding mother to rest and recover from pregnancy and childbirth. The hormones ensure that the nutrients that she gave to her baby during pregnancy are replenished. In the long term these changes are associated with a decrease in the mother's risk for diabetes and perhaps other problems yet to be discovered by medical research.

- Protectiveness. The hormones of lactation are associated with bonding, a feeling of connection between the mother and her baby. Many mothers feel protective as well. This is important and normal. Overseeing a baby's welfare is important because human babies are fragile and depend on their parents for survival.

Don't think that the way you feel is unimportant. Talk over your breastfeeding experience with your healthcare provider, especially if you're feeling sad, tired, or worried.

30. How much milk does a baby get at each breastfeeding?

Babies do not receive the same amount of milk every time. Women have different capacities for storing milk in their breasts. This is not related to the size of the breasts but rather to the amount of space inside them that milk can expand into before giving the milk cells the message to slow milk production and make less milk.

In addition, thriving babies take different amounts of milk at different feedings and stop when they have had enough. When young babies are bottle fed, they are obligated to keep swallowing as long as the milk keeps flowing. This often leads to overfeeding.

Your breastfeeding care provider can estimate how much milk a baby is transferring by weighing the baby in the same clothes and diaper before and after nursing using a digital scale accurate to 2 grams.

Should a breastfed baby lose weight?

Babies lose weight at first because of fluids they still have from being inside their mother. They're expected to lose around 7% of body weight. If they lose more than 7%, breastfeeding may have got off to a slow start, or there may be some other issue with feeding or the baby's condition that needs to be resolved.

The American Academy of Pediatrics[3] recommends the following schedule as a minimum for formal individualized breastfeeding assessments:

- Two times a day in the hospital or birth center
- At 3–5 days of age
- At 2–3 weeks by the pediatrician
- More often if the baby is having breastfeeding issues

How much should a baby gain?

As a general rule, babies double their birth weight by 6 months and triple their birth weight by a year. Breastfed babies are leaner at a year than formula-fed babies, but they gain faster in the early months.

---

[3]American Academy of Pediatrics. (2005). Breastfeeding and the use of human milk. *Pediatrics, 115*(2), 496–506.

Can a breastfed baby gain too much?

If the baby is being exclusively breastfed in the first 6 months, we don't think the baby can be overfed. However, when plotted on growth charts developed from populations of largely formula-fed infants, exclusively breastfed infants *seem* to be gaining too much in the early months and not enough in the later months of the 1st year. So it's best to plot breastfed babies on charts that have been developed for them.

PART THREE

The Breastfeeding Experience

How will I know when to feed my baby and when to end feedings?

If I'm breastfeeding, how can I take time away from my baby?

How can I safely store expressed millk?

More ...

31. It seems as if all I do is feed, change, and comfort my baby. Is that what life is like for breastfeeding mothers?

The reality of life with a baby is quite different than you may have imagined before your baby's birth. Newborn babies seem to have no apparent schedule to their lives. Like many new parents, you may be frustrated by the seemingly endless cycle of feeding, changing, and comforting your baby. You may wonder when you'll get to sleep through the night, indulge in a relaxing shower or bath, or have a few moments to rest and relax by yourself. Don't worry, your life will settle into a more predictable pattern soon.

Because of their tiny stomach capacity, newborn babies need to feed 10–12 times in 24 hours. However, most babies don't feed every 2–2.4 hours. Most babies favor a feeding pattern in which several feedings are clustered close together (this is called "cluster feeding"), they get a few hours of sleep, and then they awaken to start the frequent feedings again. To feed your baby adequately, offer the breast when your baby shows feeding cues. These signals (listed in Table 3) indicate a desire for food.

Because of their tiny stomach capacity, newborn babies need to feed 10–12 times in 24 hours.

The best way to observe these signals is to have your baby close to you. In the early days after birth, it's best to hold the baby in your arms, skin to skin, as much as possible. Not only will it be easier to rest and observe the baby for feeding cues this way, but also studies show that babies demonstrate more feeding cues when they're able to smell and hear their mothers.

Once you observe feeding cues, feed the baby as soon as possible. All you need are clean hands. It's not necessary to change the baby or do other cleaning activities before feeding.

What about night feedings?

Typically, young babies are unable to sleep for more than 5 straight hours in a 24-hour time period. If that 5-hour period happens during the day, it cannot be repeated at night—babies just don't have the stomach capacity to take in enough food for more sleep. Eventually, babies' stomachs grow, and they can consume more milk per feeding so that they can sleep for longer periods. For most babies, this happens around 4 months of age.

How can I feed so often without getting exhausted?

If your baby is near you, it should be relatively easy to feed on cue. During the day, many mothers use slings or other soft baby carriers to hold their babies. Many slings are designed to allow the baby to nurse while the mother is involved in other activities, such as cooking, reading, cleaning, working, caring for older children, etc.

The American Academy of Pediatrics[4] recommends that at night your baby sleep in the same room as you, close by. If your baby sleeps in a crib, cradle, or cobedding unit right next to your bed, it's easy to scoop up the baby and feed with little disruption. Many mothers are scarcely aware of the number of times their baby feeds at night because it can be quite restful. Perhaps your baby sleeps with you in a family bed. This is also compatible with feeding, as long as you observe safe sleep practices. (See Question 48 for more about this topic.)

---

[4]American Academy of Pediatrics. (2005). Breastfeeding and the use of human milk. *Pediatrics, 115*(2), 496–506.

32. Can I feed too often?

It never hurts to offer your baby the breast when you see feeding cues, even if it has been only a few minutes since the last feeding. Breast milk is very easy to digest, so your baby may want to fill up again within an hour of feeding.

As discussed earlier, young babies should feed at least 10 to 12 times per 24-hour time period. Just like adults, they rarely feed at regular intervals. Think about everything you ate and drank in the past 24 hours. Were your meals and snacks evenly distributed over that time period? Or did you sometimes have a drink, snack (even a stick of gum), or dessert within an hour or so of a meal? Like most adults, babies seem to prefer a schedule of several snacks and meals per day.

If you feel as if your baby is never satisfied, it's a good idea to have a skilled breastfeeding care provider observe a feeding or two. Your care provider may be able to suggest ways to improve breastfeeding positioning or latching so that your baby is able to get as much milk as he or she wants per feeding.

Does feeding frequency change as babies get older?

After 4 months of age, babies may require fewer feedings per day; however, most babies will feed 8 or more times per day during the first 6 months.

33. Should feedings always take the same amount of time?

In the first few days of life, babies may spend 20–30 minutes at the breast. This is probably for two reasons:

(1) the first milk, colostrum, is sticky, thick, and more difficult to remove and (2) the newborn baby needs practice to become a good feeder. After the first 4 days of life, babies become more adept at nursing, and milk composition changes as the second stage of milk making begins. This often means that babies will nurse for only 10–15 minutes per feeding.

If feedings routinely take more than 20 minutes after the 3rd day of life, a skilled breastfeeding care provider should evaluate a feeding. Your breastfeeding care provider may be able to help you fine-tune breastfeeding positioning and latch to improve the rate of milk flow.

34. How will I know when to feed my baby and when to end feedings?

The signs that babies are hungry include the feeding cues in Table 3. Please note that crying is not on this list. Unfortunately, many people wait for babies to cry before feeding them. Crying is a difficult state for babies. In this state their stress hormone levels are high, and they are much too upset to learn new activities, such as breastfeeding.

When your baby is very upset and crying, the best thing to do is to soothe the baby by skin-to-skin contact, rocking, walking, quiet singing, reducing the noise and brightness of the environment, etc. This is not the time to force the baby to the breast. In fact, babies who have been forced to the breast while they're crying may refuse the breast at the next feeding.

When should I end a feeding?

Ideally, you shouldn't end the feeding—the baby should. When a baby has received enough milk, his stomach is stretched, and his gastrointestinal organs begin to produce hormones. These hormones relax the baby. You can view this phenomenon by looking for the fullness cues listed in Table 6.

What if my baby falls asleep as soon as he attaches to the breast?

This sometimes happens with newborn and premature babies. The best thing to do is keep them stripped down to their diaper and hold them skin to skin with you (with blankets or clothes over the two of you as needed for your physical comfort and the baby's head out from under the covers). When babies are skin to skin with their mothers, they're more alert. Swaddled babies and those who are too warmly dressed may attach to the nipple and go back to sleep. Keeping your baby skin to skin with you increases the sensory input to the baby's nerves, which makes it more likely that he will continue feeding.

If your baby falls asleep early in the feeding, you can try massaging the breast when the baby stops suckling.

Table 6   Fullness Cues

- The baby releases the breast.
- The baby's eyes relax and facial muscles soften.
- The baby's body tone softens, fists uncurl, and arms and legs relax.
- The baby smiles or lolls his head.
- The baby makes satisfied sounds.
- The baby is drowsy or falls asleep.

Gently massaging the area around the areola will often move some milk down to the baby, encouraging the baby to stay awake and feed.

If you're unable to keep your baby awake at the breast for more than a few feedings, contact a breastfeeding care provider. Having a feeding observation may help identify ways to fine-tune breastfeeding so that it works better for you and your baby.

What if I need to end the feeding?

Although it's ideal for the baby to end the feeding, there are times when you need to stop a feeding (such as when you're in pain or when the doorbell rings). To end the feeding, place your clean finger in the corner of the baby's lips, and wait until the baby releases the seal on your breast. Alternatively, you can use your fingers to (gently) press your breast to the opposite corner of the baby's mouth. Once the seal of the baby's lips and tongue to the breast is broken, you can remove your breast from the mouth. Please don't just pull it out—that can cause trauma to the breast! Babies can generate more suction than you might think!

35. What if it hurts to breastfeed?

If it hurts to breastfeed, something is amiss. It could be that your baby is not correctly positioned or latched on. Review the guidance for positioning and latch in Questions 21 and 22. You may have some damage to your nipples. In this case read the guidance in Question 75 and Table 7 for help with deciphering the source of your pain. If the suggestions in these sections do not help you feed comfortably, please seek help. Many people think that it's normal for breastfeeding to hurt. We disagree! When feeding hurts, it's a signal to get help. Find a skilled breastfeeding care provider, and request a feeding observation.

36. My baby doesn't take the second breast at some feedings. Will the baby get enough milk from only one breast per feeding?

Many babies feed on only one breast per feeding. Whether your baby needs one breast or two at each feeding is specific to you and your baby. Some women have large, fast-flowing milk supplies, and babies can remove enough milk in 5 minutes or less to satisfy them. Other mothers have less milk in reserve, and their babies may need to nurse on each side for 20 minutes total or more per feeding. Studies show that the internal milk storage capacity of breasts varies widely from woman to woman and has no association with the external size of the breast. How much milk you can make and store between feedings depends on your breasts' milk storage capacity.

Bottom line: One breast or two per feeding is absolutely fine. As long as your baby finishes the feeding on her own and demonstrates two or more fullness cues (see Table 6) at the end of the feeding, then she has most likely taken as much milk as she needs at this feeding. If you're not certain that she took enough milk, you can offer her the second breast. If she doesn't want to nurse, she's probably full—at least for the next few minutes!

The Breastfeeding Experience

Table 7 Breast/Pain Problems

Characteristic	When	Possible reasons	Other symptoms	Things to try	If no resolution
Nipple pain throughout the feeding	Pain throughout the feeding	Latch	Could also experience shoulder pain or tension during feeding.	Go back and reexamine the baby's latch.	Pain should resolve by correcting latch.
Nipple pain in the first couple of seconds	Pain only in the first few seconds	The baby may not be initially latching correctly, but when the milk begins to flow, the baby's position changes slightly.	None	Watch the baby during the feeding. What does the position look like when the pain is gone? Try to latch the baby from that position from the start of the next feeding (his head may be tilted differently).	Pain should resolve by correcting latch.
Pain deep in the breast	During nursing	Bacterial infection	None	Call your healthcare provider, who may prescribe antibiotic therapy and anti-inflammatory drugs.	Ultrasound imaging can rule out an abscess.
Burning pain	During and after a feeding	A yeast infection (also called "candida" or "thrush")	There may be white patches in the baby's mouth. The mother may have shiny, flaky skin on the nipple and areola.	Call your healthcare provider as well as the baby's, who may prescribe antifungal drugs. Mother, baby, and any potentially contaminated items must be treated. These can include breast pump parts, pacifiers,	If the prescriptions for the mother and baby are not working, look for other things that could harbor yeast. The mother and baby's healthcare provider may try a

different antifungal prescription. If there's no sign of yeast in the baby and burning pain in the mother, the baby's incorrect latch could be causing the burning pain.

bottle nipples, and any other object that can harbor candida. In some cases, another family member may harbor candida. Treatment is only effective when the infection has been eliminated on other contaminated items and in other family members.

In addition, breast pump parts, washable breast pads, bras, and other possibly contaminated items should be carefully cleaned. The usual recommendation is to boil any components that touch the skin or the milk for 20 minutes or to soak them for several hours in the vinegar solution described above. Be sure to rinse well with clean water. Pacifiers are best discarded.

continues

The Breastfeeding Experience

Table 7   Breast/Pain Problems   *(continued)*

Characteristic	When	Possible reasons	Other symptoms	Things to try	If no resolution
Pain involving cracks or scabs on the nipple	Pain in the beginning or throughout the feeding	Cracks and scabs are caused by incorrect latch. Even with nipple trauma, there should be little to no pain when correctly latching.	The scabs and cracks may be painful throughout the day and when removing bra/clothing.	Work on latch. Have a breastfeeding specialist observe a feeding. The baby's care provider should be asked to check the mouth, tongue, lips, and palate.	Discuss with your healthcare provider possible prescriptions for healing possible wounds. May be an infection is keeping the nipple from healing.
Nipple pain after feedings and when cold/getting out of the shower	When the baby comes off of the breast and the wet nipple gets cold, the nipple turns white and the pain is excruciating.	Do you have a family history of Raynaud's symptoms or a vasospasm/circulation issue? Raynaud's can possibly develop from nipple trauma as well.	Nipple may turn white, blue, purple, pink.	Warming the nipple immediately after the baby latches off Avoiding caffeine and nicotine Carefully latching on and latching off	Talk to your healthcare provider. Drug treatment has been prescribed with success.
If the nipple appears creased or misshapen	When the baby comes off the breast, the nipple looks compressed, like a new lipstick.	Did it happen from the start or when your milk came in? If it happened from the start, the baby is probably not latching correctly. If it happened when your milk came in, the baby could be	A white line and blisters may develop along the crease. Even if there's some blood in the	Check that you're bringing the baby to breast (not directing the nipple to the baby) and that the baby's head is able to slightly tilt back during the latch. Try the semireclined or Australian posture to use gravity to help control the flow.	A few babies exert higher-than-average pressure against the breast; others may have palate shapes that require persistent corrective measures. The arrival of abundant milk flow may

	trying to slow down the flow.	encourage some babies to decrease pressure. "Tongue tie" may be associated with continuous sore nipples. Many mothers have reported relief after the frenulum stretches or has been separated by a qualified healthcare provider.	
The nipple has cracks, fissures, could be bleeding	The nipple face or sides of the nipple are cracked and may bleed	Cracks and fissures on the nipple are practically all caused from latching difficulties. Other kinds of sores may require immediate assessment from your healthcare provider.	Correcting the latch should lead to immediate pain relief during nursing. Even if the nipple has severe trauma, the pain during breastfeeding will be minimal. A small amount of pain may be present during nursing for a day or two. Resting the nipple and pumping for a few days does not guarantee relief because the root of the issue is incorrect latch and the baby needs the chance to correct the latch.
		milk, it's still OK for the baby	See your healthcare provider if nipple cracks do not heal. There may be a topical infection.

continues

The Breastfeeding Experience

Table 7   Breast/Pain Problems   *(continued)*

Characteristic	When	Possible reasons	Other symptoms	Things to try	If no resolution
Nipple pain that radiates through the breast and even to the back	A firm, small, white spot (bleb, or duct blocked near the nipple pore opening) of accumulated milk solids visible on the nipple face	The mother experiences nipple pain while the baby is latched on and actively nursing as well as in between breastfeedings. Pain usually also increases when anything (such as clothing) touches the breast.	Bleb (sometimes called a "milk blister")	Try soaking the breast in warm water before nursing or hand expression to help loosen the bleb. Examine possible reasons for the bleb: Why did the bleb form? Is part of the breast draining poorly? Is it a tight bra? Underwire? Other constriction on milk flow? Bruise? Was there a plugged duct further up in the breast before the bleb formed? No one really understands the reasons for blebs, so it's possible you'll not be sure of the cause.	Once the bleb and the milk behind are removed, the pain should decrease markedly. Occasionally, mothers find they need a surgeon to lance the bleb. It's a very fast, often in the office, procedure. Breastfeeding can then continue.

The Breastfeeding Experience

Common Breast problems

Issue	Characteristic	When	Possible reasons	Other symptoms	Things to try	If no resolution
Plugged ducts, caked breast	Hard, red tender area of the breast	Can happen at any point in lactation	Lack of milk moving from that area or pressure on that area of the breast (from carrying a diaper bag or from the seam or underwire of a bra)	None	Improve flow, avoid pressure, gentle hand expression	Call your healthcare provider if the lump doesn't move and disappear in 24–48 hours.
Mastitis	Red streaks on the breast with fever	Can happen at any point in lactation	May have also had incorrect latch and nipple trauma; may have allowed too much time between nursings	Fever, sudden aching all over	Call your healthcare provider for possible antibiotic therapy and anti-inflammatory drugs.	Recurrent mastitis is associated with anemia.
Mastitis in both breasts	Red streaks on both breasts with fever	More likely in the early time postpartum	Systemic strep infection (unrelated to breastfeeding)	Fever, delirium, aching all over	Immediately call your healthcare provider and go to the emergency room.	
Abscess	Pus-filled lump in the breast that does not move	Often after mastitis	May be an unresolved aspect of mastitis	None	Medical evaluation Bed rest and continued breastfeeding Continued breastfeeding on the affected side, if possible. If putting the baby to the breast is not possible, use hand	Go to your healthcare provider, who will probably refer you to a surgeon. The worst solution is to stop breastfeeding/milk expression

continues

Table 7 Breast/Pain Problems (continued)

Issue	Characteristic	When	Possible reasons	Other symptoms	Things to try	If no resolution
					expression or gentle pumping to remove milk.	altogether or even stopping only on the affected side. Suddenly stopping breastfeeding will make the problem worse by adding engorgement to the problem. Drain or surgically remove the abscess. Sometimes the physician is able to use a needle to reduce the lump. The newer technique is to use ultrasound to insert a drain (or drains). Often surgery is performed in an outpatient setting with local anesthesia. The incision should be made as far away from the nipple and areola as possible. Every attempt should be made to avoid cutting across ducts.

Issue	Characteristic	Reasons	Possible impact on breastfeeding	Possible resolution
Engorgement	Painfully swollen breasts	Often between day 2 and 4 after birth, but can happen anytime in the early weeks if the baby is not feeding often or effectively enough. The baby is not removing a sufficient amount of milk from the breast.	Nipple may appear tight or flat because of the amount of milk tightening the skin. Nipple soreness can occur if the breast is so full that the baby has difficulty latching.	Increase frequency and efficiency of breastfeedings. Relieve pressure and pain by allowing excess milk to flow out of the breast. Water is a wonderful aid—take a shower or a bath, or soak your breasts in warm water to help the milk flow and to relieve compression. Consult your healthcare provider.
Anemia	Low iron levels in mother's blood	Chronic anemia, anemia due to blood loss during or after the birth of your baby, and or other medical issues that can lead to anemia	Anemia-related breastfeeding problems may relate to the anemia itself or to the fact that the mother is too tired to put her baby to the breast frequently enough. Recurrent mastitis may hapapen more in anemic women.	Blood iron levels increase to normal.

continues

The Breastfeeding Experience

Table 7 Breast/Pain Problems (continued)

Issue	Characteristic	Reasons	Possible impact on breastfeeding	Possible resolution
Thyroid problems	Hyperthyroidism Hypothyroidism	It could be a disorder that the mother had before pregnancy or birth, or it could be a new issue.	Disorders related to the thyroid can impact milk production.	Thyroid levels are normalized with medications or medical intervention.
Sheehan's syndrome	Blood loss, dull dry hair, copious hair loss, milk supply issues	Significant loss during the birth, which affects the mother's pituitary gland	Decreased milk supply because of the damage to the pituitary	The mother may decide to put the baby to breast and feed the baby milk from a milk bank or formula through an at-breast supplementer.
Postpartum depression	Tired, sad (see Edinburgh Postpartum Depression Scale in Table 11).	Postpartum mood disturbance	If your healthcare provider prescribes antidepressants, there are many options that are compatible with breastfeeding.	Antidepressants, therapy

37. If I'm breastfeeding, how can I take time away from my baby?

In the early days postpartum, it's best to stay in contact with your baby as much as possible. Before your baby was born, your body helped regulate many of your baby's body systems. Your heart pushed blood containing oxygen, nutrients, and hormones to your baby's placenta. Your heartbeat became the rhythmic background of your baby's life. After birth, your baby relies on listening to your heartbeat, hearing your breathing, and sensing your presence to help adapt to independent life on earth. Babies who are held in skin-to-skin contact with their mother's body have more normal heart rates, breathing rates, and better oxygen levels in their blood.

However, after the first weeks of life, many mothers long for a few moments by themselves. Perhaps you're longing for a walk around the block, a quick trip to the store, or a massage or bubble bath. Taking some time for yourself can be beneficial and can certainly be compatible with breastfeeding.

After the first few weeks of life, many babies settle into predictable feeding and sleeping patterns. If this happens with your baby, you'll have a good sense of what time of day is best to plot your getaway. Arrange for your partner, a family member, or a friend to care for your baby during this time. You'll want to leave some expressed breast milk in case your baby should awaken and show feeding cues during your absence. See Questions 39 and 41 for information about expressing and storing milk.

Perhaps you're planning a longer period of time (e.g., a night or weekend) apart from your baby. You may be planning to build a supply of stored milk or have

Taking some time for yourself can be beneficial and can certainly be compatible with breastfeeding.

The Breastfeeding Experience

81

someone feed the baby formula during this time. Longer separation (e.g., a night or longer) can also be more psychologically difficult for you and your baby than you might think. Some babies refuse to make eye contact or to nurse after separation from their mother. Some babies are overjoyed to be reunited with their mother. Other babies are upset and clingy after prolonged separation from their mother.

Many women find that although they look forward to having some time for themselves, they spend much of the time away from their baby thinking about and worrying about their baby. This is normal. There is no reason to force yourself to stay apart from your baby if you find yourself not enjoying the break.

38. Should I feed my baby with a bottle at times when I can't breastfeed?

You've probably heard about breastfed babies who refused to accept a bottle. Perhaps you've heard that you should start your breastfed baby on a bottle right away so that he won't refuse it later. This may seem to make sense, but research does not support this practice. Research shows that suckling is involuntary until the baby is several weeks of age. So a very young baby will suckle on a bottle nipple placed in his mouth, even if he isn't hungry. But, once he reaches 2 months of age, the same baby may refuse the bottle, even if he accepted it earlier. So there is no need to introduce bottles to your healthy breastfeeding newborn. The vast majority of babies need nothing in the first 6 months of life but their mother's milk. In rare cases where a woman does not make enough milk or where the baby has a medical need for formula, formula may be given to the baby.

What's the best way to give a supplement to a breastfed baby?

There's no simple answer to this question. If a woman is trying to build her milk supply, her breastfeeding helper may recommend the use of an at-breast feeder, a **nursing supplementer**. This device attaches a tube to the breast, which is fed from a container of formula or expressed breast milk that hangs around the mother's neck. With this device, the baby receives all her food at the breast, and the increased suckling time may help the mother's body produce more milk.

When babies are born prematurely, have heart conditions, or are ill, they may be unable to suckle strongly enough to stimulate the production of adequate milk. In this case the baby may be supplemented with a small cup. This method of feeding appears to be less stressful for these babies than feeding with the bottle. In this event parents will be taught how to feed their baby with a cup (it's somewhat different from the method we use to cup-feed ourselves).

Perhaps the baby is unable to suckle effectively at the breast, as in the case of a baby with Down syndrome, a **cleft palate**, or other medical condition affecting the strength or integrity of the baby's mouth. In this case the baby may be supplemented with special spoons, tubes, bottles with uncommonly shaped nipples, or other devices to accommodate her abilities to feed. For more information about these special situations, see the questions in Part 7.

Nursing supplementer
fine plastic tubing, with one end attached to a container holding expressed human milk or formula and the other end taped to the breast

Cleft palate
a congenital birth defect causing a division or opening in the roof of the mouth

What about pacifiers?

Studies have shown that mothers stop breastfeeding earlier when they give their babies pacifiers frequently. Babies who use pacifiers often have fewer feedings per day. Why? Perhaps some mothers offer pacifiers when their babies show feeding cues. While the baby is suckling on the pacifier, he's not stimulating his mother's milk-making hormones. Not surprisingly, excessive pacifier use can decrease a woman's ability to make milk.

But I've heard that pacifiers decrease the risk of sudden infant death syndrome (SIDS). Is that true?

SIDS

sudden infant death syndrome—see **crib death**

Crib death

the unexpected and sudden death, of unknown origin, of a seemingly normal and healthy infant that occurs during sleep; also called "sudden infant death syndrome," or SIDS

Sudden infant death syndrome (**SIDS**) is the name for a syndrome in which babies under 1 year of age die for unknown reasons. It's also called **crib death** because SIDS victims are often found dead in their cribs.

In 2005, the American Academy of Pediatrics (AAP) made a list of recommendations for reducing the number of SIDS deaths. Among these was a suggestion that parents consider offering their babies a pacifier at nap and bedtime (research has indicated a decreased risk of SIDS with pacifier use). As part of this recommendation, the AAP stated that pacifiers should not be offered to exclusively breastfed babies until 1 month of age (to allow breastfeeding to become well established).

Currently, there is controversy about the science behind this recommendation to offer all babies pacifiers. It appears that the babies at greatest risk for SIDS are those who always use a pacifier to transition to sleep but who don't have it on the day of their death (e.g., because they're sleeping away from home or because the pacifier has been lost). It's not clear whether the pacifier's presence protects the baby or whether the usual pacifier's absence poses a greater risk for SIDS.

If you introduce pacifiers, it's best to use them sparingly. Babies who use pacifiers regularly appear to have higher risk of ear infection.

It's up to you to determine whether you offer a pacifier to your baby. But it's best to avoid using pacifiers until breastfeeding is well established, and breastfeeding reduces the risk of SIDS. Familiarize yourself with the AAP's other recommendations for SIDS reduction, including the following: putting the baby to sleep on his back; using a firm, safe sleep surface; keeping soft objects (pillows, stuffed animals, duvets, etc.) out of the sleep space; avoiding smoking during pregnancy and after birth; putting the baby to sleep in a separate crib or cot that is close to your bed; avoiding overdressing the baby for sleep; avoiding commercial devices designed to reduce SIDS; avoiding use of home monitors to decrease SIDS; avoiding flattening the baby's head by offering tummy time frequently when the baby is awake and decreasing time spent in upright positions (in car seats, bouncer seats, etc.); and making sure that all child care providers and babysitters are aware of these ways to reduce the risk of SIDS.

39. How can I remove my milk to be fed to the baby when we're separated?

Removing (also called "expressing") your milk for your baby is a great way to continue the benefits of breastfeeding when you're not with your baby. If you haven't given birth yet, ask your nurse or breastfeeding helper to show you how to remove milk from your breast after your baby is born. Your first milk (colostrum) will be sticky and thick, and you may only collect a few drops. This is normal. When your mature milk comes in around the 3rd day after birth, the composition of the milk will help you collect more.

Even if you plan to use a breast pump to collect milk, you should learn to express milk by hand (this is also called "manual expression"). This method of milk removal is always available to you, needs no electricity or special equipment, and helps stimulate the hormones that control milk production and removal. At first, you may remove less than an ounce of milk. As your technique improves and your milk supply increases, you'll collect more milk. Don't lose confidence in your milk supply based on what you can express from your breast. Babies are much more efficient at milk removal than any device or technique. One technique for hand expression is described in Table 8. (See also Figure 21.)

40. How can I determine which breast pump is best for me?

There's no easy answer to this question. Women like different pumps for varying reasons. It's important to take several factors into consideration when choosing a pump:

- How much milk you need to remove. If you're pumping for a premature or sick baby, a rental-grade pump with automatic double-pumping ability is probably best. This type of pump is associated with the highest milk yield. You may also want to consider this type of pump if you will be returning to work full-time and plan to continue exclusively

Table 8   Hand Expression of Breast Milk

- Wash your hands.
- Have a clean container ready to collect the milk. The newer you are to hand expression, the wider the container should be, so start with a large lightweight bowl for the first few expressions.
- Lightly massage your breast right down to your nipple. Give your nipple a little stretch to get the hormones flowing.
- Place your thumb and index finger on your areola (the dark circle around the nipple). Push back toward your chest wall, and then compress your thumb and finger together gently. It's best if you don't slide your fingers on your skin. Some women like to use a rolling motion.
- Position the collecting container on a table if you're standing up or on your lap if you're sitting down. Try to aim the spray into the container.
- Repeat the push back and compress gently motion in the same place on your breast until the flow slows down.
- Move the finger and thumb to another spot, and repeat.
- Switch to the other breast. When you get comfortable with this, you may be able to express both breasts at the same time, but you will probably need two bowls!

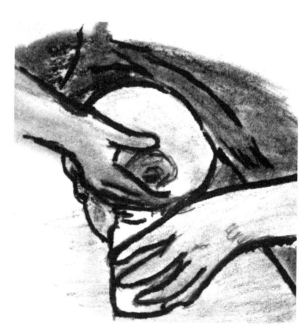

Figure 21   Hand Expression
Hand expression is one way to remove milk from your breasts.

The Breastfeeding Experience

breastfeeding. However, if you're planning to express milk for an occasional relief bottle, this type of pump is not necessary.

- How often you plan to pump. If you plan to pump multiple times daily, be sure that your pump is comfortable and built for heavy use. If you plan to pump once daily or less, any of the smaller manual pumps may work fine and be very cost effective.

- How much you want to spend. Pumps cost between $10 and $1,000. If you plan to use the pump multiple times daily for many months, calculate the cost of a rental-grade pump versus a retail pump. In many situations renting may be less expensive than purchasing.

- Whether you have an electric power source available. Some electric motor pumps have adaptors for use in an automobile. If you don't have access to electricity in the locations you'll be pumping, consider a battery pack or battery-operated pump. Battery-operated pumps may continue to make noise but not function effectively when the batteries are not fully charged. You may want to consider purchasing rechargeable batteries to decrease costs.

- How involved you want to be in the pumping. Pumps can be manually operated (requiring hand squeezing or pulling a piston) or fully automatic (requiring you to just hold the pump shield to your breasts).

- Whether you want to pump one or two breasts at a time. Double pumping is associated with increased milk collection but often requires you to have both hands free. Many women like to pump with one hand free so they can multitask.

Take some time to shop around for the best pump for your situation.

The US Food and Drug Administration maintains a Web site (see Appendix) to help you choose a pump. You'll also find complaints and recalls on this Web site. It's a good idea to check here for complaints about the pump you're considering purchasing. Also, keep these tips in mind:

- Before buying an electric or battery-operated pump, ask the manufacturer the expected motor life of the pump you're considering. Some pumps that cost hundreds of dollars have very limited motor life. Some women buy these more expensive pumps expecting to use those pumps for several babies, only to discover they've exceeded the motor life with the first baby. When the motor ages, the pump may still make noise but not function as efficiently. If the volume of milk you're expressing suddenly decreases after weeks or months of pumping, have your pump checked out.

- Don't use secondhand pumps—only rental-grade pumps should be used by more than one user. Pumps sold on the retail market are intended for only one user. The motors of these pumps can become contaminated and spread infection from one mother to another. Used pumps bought at yard sales, found on the Internet, or borrowed from a friend can transmit herpes, hepatitis, and other diseases from one mother to another mother's baby.

- When using a rental pump, be sure that you're using your own pumping kit. All the pieces of the pump that touch your breast and your milk should be new for you and used only by you!

- Use and clean your breast pump according to the manufacturer's instructions. A list of pump company Web sites and other information appears in the Appendix.

The Breastfeeding Experience

- Be sure to read your pump's instructions fully and to ask for help with use, if needed. Incorrect use can hurt and damage your breast tissue.
- Don't use parts from one company on another company's pumps.

For specific information about locating pumps, please see the resource list in the Appendix.

41. How can I safely store expressed milk?

If you're collecting milk for a premature, fragile, ill, or hospitalized baby, please ask your nurse or doctor for specific milk storage instructions.

For some babies, the milk must be frozen. In other cases, the milk should not be frozen or warmed so that all the components of human milk are preserved. If the baby is hospitalized, you may need to store and freeze the milk in the same small quantities that the baby is being fed.

If you're storing milk for a healthy baby, consider the following tips:

- You should store your milk in the amount that you're going to give the baby at one feeding, not in the amount that you have expressed. When your baby is small, it's best to store milk in 1- or 2-ounce amounts. Why? Because a baby's stomach capacity is small, and any milk left over after a feeding must be discarded. You don't want 3 ounces of your hard work going down the drain!

- Reusable glass or hard-sided plastic containers are considered the best for storing breast milk. It's important that the cap fits securely. The same companies that make pumps and other equipment make milk storage containers. In addition, some food-packaging companies—for example, Snappies™ and Mother's Milkmate™—make hard-sided containers specifically for breast milk. You may also use other hard-sided plastic food storage containers (e.g., Tupperware® and Rubbermaid®) with tight lids as well as small glass jars (such as baby food jars).
- You may also buy plastic bags that have been specifically manufactured to collect and store mother's milk. Some of these can be pumped into; the bags may be used to store and feed as well. Handle carefully—they can be awkward to manage and can leak.
- Each container of milk should be labeled at least with the date. When a baby is premature or hospitalized for any reason, the hospital will either give the mother labels for her milk or tell her specific information that she should put on the label, including the date, the patient ID number, unit, etc. If you're taking the milk to a day care setting, write the baby's name legibly with a waterproof, smudge-proof marker.

How long can I safely store milk?

We asked international milk expert Lois D. W. Arnold, PhD, this question, and she developed the algorithm in Figure 22. You may notice that her suggestions are more conservative than some others you may see; that's because they're public health recommendations based on the evidence and aimed at keeping milk at the highest possible quality.

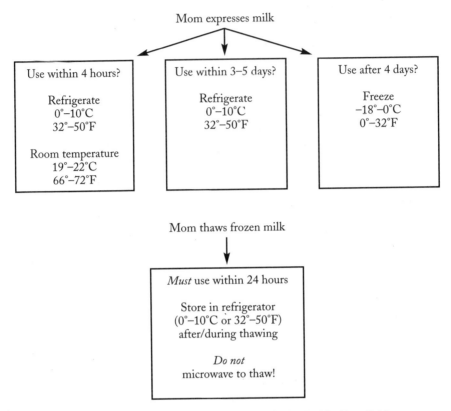

Figure 22   Algorithm for Storage of Expressed Breast Milk for Healthy-Term Babies

To use the algorithm in Figure 22, ask yourself, "How soon do I need to use the milk?" Other guidelines to follow include these:

You can safely store milk for 3–5 days in the refrigerator.

- You can safely store milk for 3–5 days in the refrigerator. But, if you're going to freeze it, put it in the freezer as soon as you can.
- You can keep milk up to 3 months in a refrigerator freezer and up to 6 months in a deep freeze that is kept at -20°F or less.
- Over the course of a day, you can add small expressions of milk to milk stored in the refrigerator. The new milk must be chilled before being added to milk that is already cold.

- The coldest part of the refrigerator or freezer is the best place to keep milk. That's usually not on the door or near the fan in a frost-free freezer.

How can I thaw and reheat my stored milk?

- Always thaw frozen breast milk in the container in which it was frozen.
- Defrost frozen milk in the refrigerator.
- Warm refrigerated or frozen milk in a pan of luke-warm water or under lukewarm running tap water.
- Never use a microwave to thaw or warm breast milk or any other baby foods. Babies have been burned because of hot spots that were not detectable by the adult. Breast milk is especially vulnerable to micro-waves, which can damage milk components.
- Keep thawed breast milk cold until just before feeding it to the baby.
- Use thawed breast milk within 24 hours of defrosting it.
- Do not refreeze thawed breast milk.

What does expressed milk look like?

You may be surprised by the way your milk looks. During pregnancy and immediately after birth, your milk looks thick and very yellowish (almost orange, sometimes). Why? Because of the high levels of immune factors in this early milk, which offer great protection to your baby.

As milk changes from colostrum to mature milk, it becomes creamy in color and finally blue-white. Many women look at their mature milk and think it looks weak or like skim milk. It's not weak at all—it's the perfect food for human babies!

When you store expressed milk in the refrigerator, it will separate—the fat will rise to the top of the container. This is normal. It does not mean the milk has gone bad. When using the milk, gently shake the container to resuspend the fat in the milk.

Women sometimes report that after milk has been frozen, it has a sour or rancid smell. This seems to happen because active enzymes in the milk break down fat as the milk is freezing. You can offer this milk to your baby as long as it has been safely stored (see information earlier in Question 41). If your baby refuses this sour-smelling milk, you may want to get in the habit of scalding the milk (heating your milk in a pan until bubbles appear on the surface of the fluid) and then immediately freezing it. This seems to stop the action of the enzymes without losing much of the nutrients in your milk.

Sometimes women express milk that is red, brown, pink, or green in color. This may happen after you eat a lot of a strongly colored food or drink or as a harmless side effect of a medication. Red or brown in the milk can also be blood. It's not a problem for the baby to drink milk with blood in it—milk is made from blood that circulates to the milk-making cells, after all. However, when you see signs of blood in your milk, you should see your breastfeeding care provider or primary care provider to have the source of the bleeding evaluated. Most often this comes from unhealed nipple trauma. Please be sure to get help with breastfeeding so your nipples can heal.

42. I'm worried about being embarrassed. How can I nurse discreetly in public?

It's normal to have concerns about nursing in public. Many nursing women don't want to be embarrassed, and they don't want to embarrass others. Having said that, you've probably seen hundreds of mothers and babies nursing in public without ever being aware of what was going on. All you need to nurse discreetly is clothing that covers your side and a blanket or shawl to place over your shoulder when you're putting your baby to the breast and removing your baby from the breast. Many women find it helpful to practice discreet nursing in front of a mirror at home before venturing out.

Helpful clothing for nursing in public includes layered outfits, such as a tank top or T-shirt under an opened button-up shirt. This choice allows you to cover your side at all times. Several large department stores now carry inexpensive tank tops and camisoles for nursing mothers. These tops cover your abdomen at all times. It's more difficult to nurse discreetly when wearing a dress or single top, unless the piece is specially designed for breastfeeding.

Another option for discreet public nursing is wearing your baby in a sling or soft baby carrier that accommodates breastfeeding (some front carriers do not). Of course, to nurse a baby in a sling, you still need to wear clothing that makes your breasts easily accessible. With practice, many women find that discreet public nursing becomes second nature.

Discreet nursing can become more difficult with a baby beyond 4 months of age who may become easily distracted by sounds or sights in the environment. You may have to find a dark, quiet corner to nurse your older baby. On the other hand, if you're feeling comfortable with public nursing by that time, you're doing a public service by exposing the general public to the concept of breastfeeding. You may give others their first opportunity to observe breastfeeding and learn from the experience. Know that breastfeeding in public is your legal right in most US states and is widely practiced throughout the world. You also have the right to breastfeed in or on any Federal property (such as a national park or post office) where you have the right to be. For more information about breastfeeding rights, see the Appendix.

43. My breasts have changed. Is that normal?

It's important to keep track of how your breasts feel during the breastfeeding period. The breasts go through several changes, including:

- Changes in pregnancy include an increase in cup size; an increase in nipple sensitivity; an increase in blood flow, which causes the veins to become more visible; the darkening of the areola (the darker circle around the nipple); an increase in size and prominence of the Montgomery glands (small goose-bump-like projections on the areola that secrete a fluid that lubricates and protects the nipple area); and the production of colostrum, the first milk, which may appear as a dried yellow substance on the nipple area and/or the bra.

- Changes in the first days postpartum include increased warmth as the breast enters the second stage of milk synthesis; increased nipple sensitivity because of increased blood flow to the breast; and the growth of the nipple, which occurred during pregnancy but becomes especially obvious when the baby removes her mouth from the nipple (the nipple will be stretched two or three times its resting length).

- Around the 3rd day postpartum, the breast increases again in warmth and size with the production of mature milk. This is referred to as the mature milk "coming in." Women often feel very warm and flushed and may be weepy and moody at this time because of hormonal changes.

- **Engorgement** (or overfullness) in the breast can occur at this time, or at any other time. Engorgement in the early days postpartum is caused by an excess fluid in the breast, including milk, as well as the extra raw materials sent to the breast through the blood and lymph system to provide the components of mature milk.

- Engorgement (see Figure 23) after the first days postpartum may indicate inadequate milk removal. Sometimes this happens when feedings have been missed (as often happens at holiday times and the first time the baby sleeps through the night). Other times engorgement happens because the breast is making more milk than the baby is taking (this may occur when the milk supply is very abundant or the baby experiences discomfort, such as an ear infection or teething, that makes it difficult to sustain feeding). Part of the breast may become engorged because clothing constricts the flow of milk through that area. Whenever engorgement occurs, it's important to identify the cause. Prolonged engorgement can lead

Engorgement
swelling in the breast that blocks milk flow, caused by inadequate or infrequent milk removal; the breast will be hot and painful and will look tight and shiny; with severe engorgement, milk production may stop

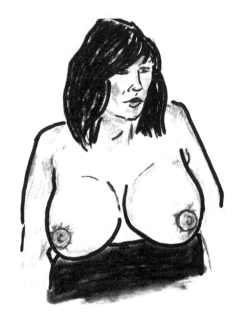

Figure 23 Engorgement
When the breasts are engorged, they're hard and hot. The skin may be so stretched that it's shiny.

Mastitis

inflammation in the breast causing localized tenderness, redness, and heat; mothers with mastitis may have a fever or headache and may feel tired, achy, or nauseous; mastitis may or may not be caused by an infection

Inflammation

a localized reaction of tissue to the presence of items perceived to be foreign or another irritation, injury, or infection that is characterized by pain, redness, and swelling

to a reduction in milk supply. Seek the help of a breastfeeding specialist as needed. Also, see Question 77 for more information about resolving engorgement.

• Softening of the breast normally occurs around the end of the 1st month of breastfeeding. This does not reflect the loss of your milk supply—but rather your body's determination that you do not need enough milk for multiple babies (unless, of course, you have muliples!). When your body determines the amount of milk needed at this stage, it sends less fluid to the breasts to provide raw materials for milk, causing a softening sensation. The breast may also appear smaller at this time.

• Reddened areas on the breast could be a sign of clogged milk ducts or **mastitis** (**inflammation** in the breast). This occurs when milk does not flow freely through a section of the breast. Reddened areas can also occur because of rashes or infections. See Question 60 for more information about these conditions. Please seek help from your medical care provider if you have unexplained red areas on the breast.

- Many women are surprised to note that their breasts feel different from pregnancy to pregnancy and from lactation to lactation. Experienced mothers often bring in a large milk supply more quickly than expected for their second and third breastfed babies. The breasts of experienced breastfeeding mothers may also enter the final stage of milk production more rapidly. In this stage milk is made during a feeding, resulting in a lesser sense of fullness between feedings.

44. What type of bra is best for breastfeeding?

There are several factors to consider in choosing a nursing bra:

Comfort is the number one consideration for a nursing bra.

- Comfort is the number one consideration for a nursing bra. A bra should not pinch, poke, or constrict your breast in any way. Make sure that you try on bras before purchasing them. If you select a bra before the birth of your child, choose one with enough space in the cups to accommodate the swelling that will occur in the early days after birth.
- Cost is another important factor. It's best to purchase only one or two bras before your baby is born. Why? Because your breast size will change in the early days of nursing. Your breasts will initially grow larger and then reduce in size. You may want to consider purchasing a few nursing tank tops or camisoles. These tops have built-in shelf bras with slits for breastfeeding. Because they're stretchy, they

can accommodate changes in your breast size in the early days postpartum.

- Selection is increasing. Be glad that you're having babies at a time when there are options beyond white cotton bras! You can now find fashionable choices—from demure bras to leopard-print bras.
- Whatever choices you make, know that it's important to wear your bra during the daytime hours only. Some women are told that they should wear bras around the clock. This is not recommended because even a bra that fits well will constrict the breasts. If you leak excessively, consider a loose-fitting tank top for bedtime, rather than a bra.

45. What can I do about leaking?

Leaking can be annoying! Many women leak when they encounter a stimulus that triggers their milk to flow. This could be anything that reminds you subconsciously of your baby—the sound of another baby crying or cooing, the smell of baby powder, the sight of a picture of your baby. The little muscles of the pores at the end of the milk ducts are responsible for holding back the flow of milk. Some women have tighter pore muscles than others. That means that some women leak often, and others don't leak at all. There is nothing we know of that can tighten these muscles.

Some women find that leaking changes throughout the period of breastfeeding as well as between babies. So if you experience leaking, don't assume that it will always be a problem for you.

Many women find that wearing nursing pads inside their bra helps reduce the signs of leaking. Nursing pads can be purchased in either disposable or reusable forms. If you choose reusable pads, it's important to choose soft, absorbent ones made of cotton or other natural materials. Avoid any pads containing a plastic lining or other moisture barrier, which will decrease airflow around the nipple and can lead to nipple discomfort. Be sure to change pads frequently to keep the nipple area relatively dry.

If you're prone to leaking, choose dark, patterned clothing. It's harder to see the wet stains from milk on dark patterns than on light solids.

If you're aware that you're starting to leak, you may be able to temporarily stop leaking by pressing your forearms or palms firmly against your breasts.

46. When should I start my baby on formula and other foods?

According to the American Academy of Pediatrics (AAP),[5] your milk contains everything your baby needs until 6 months of age (with the exception of vitamin K, which is given at birth, and 200 milligrams of vitamin D, which should be given daily by droplets beginning in the first 2 months of life). There's no need to start formula for a healthy baby. The AAP recommends that you continue breastfeeding as long as possible—at least for the 1st year and as long thereafter as you and your baby wish. In addition, the AAP states that to decrease the risk of allergies and other negative consequences, you should delay introducing solid foods until your baby is about 6 months of age. The World Health Organization encourages that breastfeeding

[5]American Academy of Pediatrics. (2005). Breastfeeding and the use of human milk. *Pediatrics, 115*(2), 496–506.

continue until at least 2 years, with the introduction of appropriate solid foods at 6 months of age.

If you choose to add some supplemental formula before these ages, we recommend that you wait until breastfeeding is well established (unless, of course, your baby has a medical need for formula). For most mothers and babies, that would mean waiting at least 1 month. Once you begin supplementing breastfeeding with formula, your baby's chances of illness and allergy do increase, so take your family history into consideration when deciding about using formula.

Perhaps you're thinking about offering your baby a bottle of formula to determine how much milk you're making. Many mothers worry that they don't have enough milk. However, "testing" breastfeeding with a bottle of formula is not recommended. When you put a bottle nipple in their mouths, newborn babies will suck on it. Sucking is involuntary at first. Babies who have never had a bottle before will take an ounce or more before they figure out how to stop the flow of fluid from the bottle. You cannot determine how much milk you're making with this test. If you have doubts about your milk supply, please contact a breastfeeding helper, who can evaluate your milk production.

Perhaps you're thinking of offering formula to have a break from your baby. You might also consider expressing some of your milk and leaving that for your baby. Expressed milk does not increase your baby's risk of allergy or illness and is more likely to be accepted by your baby than formula.

Please see Question 70 regarding how to offer solid foods to your baby.

47. What should I do if my baby bites while breastfeeding?

You may be worried about nursing your baby after she has teeth. Most babies bring in their bottom teeth first. Because a baby's tongue covers the bottom teeth during nursing, a baby is more likely to bite her tongue than your nipple. In fact, biting with top or bottom teeth can't happen when a baby is suckling properly (because the nipple is deep in the baby's mouth and the jaw is so widely open that the teeth place little pressure on the breast). Nonetheless, your baby may bite your breast either intentionally or unintentionally. The first time the baby bites, it's most likely an accident. But your reaction may seem like a great game to the playful older baby ("I bite, and you scream; I bite, and you make crazy facial expressions," etc.). If this is the case, it's best to keep the drama of your response to a minimum, remove the baby from the breast, say something such as "Mommy is not for hurting," and end the feeding. Slapping the baby or otherwise physically punishing the baby is not recommended. Just make it clear that you do not tolerate biting. When your baby requests another feeding, feed her, but keep your eyes open for the potential of some mischief at the end of the feeding. Many babies get a little twinkle in their eyes just before they bite. You may need to stay alert to these facial expressions to end the "biting game."

Other babies bite accidentally—perhaps they're falling asleep, feel the nipple slipping out of their mouth, and react by suddenly clamping down. Or perhaps they sneeze while nursing and involuntarily bite down. In these cases, make it clear that biting is not tolerated. If you yell loudly, some babies may resist going to the breast at the next feeding. Talk to your baby; tell her it's OK to feed. Even if she doesn't understand all your words, she understands the emotions behind them.

Of course, babies experience teething pain sporadically for many days, weeks, and, in some cases, months before teeth erupt. During this period your baby may sometimes be uncomfortable when nursing, probably because the action of suckling brings more blood flow and sensation to her inflamed gums. At these times it's helpful to give a baby a cold, clean object (such as a teething ring or a frozen damp facecloth) to chew on before feeding. Chewing on these objects may temporarily numb the baby's gums. If her pain continues for many feedings, consult with your pediatric care provider.

48. When will my breastfed baby sleep through the night?

This is a good question, but it's a difficult one to answer. First off, what do you mean by "sleeping through the night"? Some parents hope to put their baby to bed at 7 p.m. and have him sleep until 7 a.m. or 8 a.m. Solid sleep lasting 12 hours or more is unlikely to happen until your baby becomes a teenager!

A more realistic expectation would be for the baby to sleep from 12 a.m. to 5 a.m. without waking. Of course, no one can guarantee what time your baby will go to sleep and awaken. However, 5 to 6 hours of uninterrupted sleep is about the most you can expect from your baby before he turns 4 months of age. Your baby's small stomach capacity requires him to wake frequently and nurse to get enough food.

If that 5- to 6-hour uninterrupted sleep period happens during the day, it cannot be repeated at night—your baby just doesn't have a large enough stomach capacity to take in enough food for more sleep. Eventually, his stomach will grow, and he will be able to consume more milk per feeding and sleep for longer periods. For most babies, this happens after 4 months of age.

You might ask how parents survive a baby's sleep schedule. Many parents learn to adapt their own sleep patterns to accommodate their baby's needs in the early months. For example, some parents work to keep their baby from taking long naps in the late afternoon and early evening. Others put their baby to bed as soon as he gets sleepy but awaken him before the mother goes to bed to work in another feeding.

What about sleeping with my baby?

Caring for a baby is exhausting! Many parents do choose to sleep with their baby to be close enough to respond to the baby's needs. The decision about sleeping with your baby is a personal choice. Certainly, throughout history, babies have slept with their mothers for warmth, comfort, and food. There is some risk to that.

The decision about sleeping with your baby is a personal choice.

The American Academy of Pediatrics recommends that your baby sleep in the same room as you at night, in close proximity to you. If your baby sleeps in a crib, cradle, or cobedding unit right next to your bed, it's easy to scoop her up and feed with little disruption. Many mothers are scarcely aware of the number of times their baby feeds at night because it can be quite restful. Perhaps your baby sleeps with you in a family bed. This is also compatible with feeding, as long as you observe safe sleep practices. Tips for safe sleep practices are listed in Table 9.

Table 9   Safe Sleep Environment for Babies

A safe sleep environment for a baby includes the following factors:

- The baby should lie on his back.
- The baby should wear an appropriate level of clothing (i.e., not be overdressed).
- There should be no pillows, thick blankets, duvets, sheepskins, thick crib bumpers, feather beds, or other items on the sleep surface near the baby that could cover his head, mouth, or nose.
- The baby should never be laid to sleep on a pillow.
- There should be no gaps between the mattress and the crib or bed frame. If the baby is sleeping in a crib, the space between the upright bars of the crib sides should be less than 2.375 inches (6 centimeters) to keep the baby from slipping between the bars.
- There should be no drapery or electrical cords, no ribbons or ties on the baby's clothing, and no other potential choking or strangulation hazards near the baby.
- The baby should not cosleep with a parent or parents who:
  - Smoke cigarettes or use tobacco
  - Are taking any medications (including prescription, over-the-counter, and recreational drugs) that make them sleepy, or who are under the influence of alcohol
  - Are very overweight
  - Have sleep apnea or other sleep disturbances
  - Are extremely tired
- The baby should also not sleep in beds with older children, pets, or other family members.
- The baby should not sleep alone in adult beds because he'll be able to move about from a very early age.
- The baby should never sleep (either alone or with someone else) on a couch, chair, recliner, or waterbed.

For information on reducing the risk of sudden infant death, see Question 38.

49. When should I stop breastfeeding? How do I stop breastfeeding?

According to the American Academy of Pediatrics (AAP), your milk contains everything your baby needs until 6 months of age (see Question 46 regarding vitamins your baby needs). The AAP recommends that you continue breastfeeding as long as possible—at least for the 1st year and as long thereafter as you and your baby wish. In addition, the AAP states that to decrease the risk of allergy and other negative consequences, you should delay introducing solid foods until your baby is about 6 months of age.

It's up to you to decide how long you choose to breastfeed. Your baby will benefit from any amount of breastfeeding. However, delaying the introduction of formula as long as possible or only using breastmilk and waiting until your baby is 6 months old to introduce solid foods are the healthiest options for your baby and for you. Many of the well-known benefits of breastfeeding (such as less breast cancer and greater postpartum weight loss for moms; fewer ear infections and gastrointestinal illness for babies) are much more likely to be experienced by mothers who exclusively breastfeed their babies until 6 months.

Perhaps this is not possible for you. No one else should judge you for how you feed your baby. Ultimately, it's your choice.

The best way to wean your baby from the breast is to stop slowly. Drop one of your baby's less favorite feedings first. Think about your baby's feeding pattern. Which feedings are her favorites? Many babies love to nurse when they're waking up from sleep and again when they're returning to sleep. Replace the dropped breastfeeding with an appropriate replacement. For the baby younger than 6 months of age, the appropriate replacement would be a bottle of expressed breast milk or formula. For the baby between 6 months and a year, a good substitute would be either an appropriate solid food or a cup or bottle of expressed breast milk or formula. For the baby older than 1 year, the appropriate replacement might be food, or it might be some special contact (e.g., reading a new book, going for a walk to the park, etc.). Then watch your baby. How did she respond to the dropped feeding and replacement? If she became more clingy or dependent, you may need to go more slowly. Continue to substitute for the feeding you dropped each day. On the other hand, if she responded well to the dropped feeding, try dropping another one.

Sometimes mothers need to wean more quickly. This could be a result of her taking a contraindicated medication or having a procedure that requires breastfeeding to stop. Always get a second opinion from a breastfeeding expert when you're told that breastfeeding must stop. Unfortunately, some healthcare providers are not aware of the excellent drug and medical resources available for breastfeeding questions—if they don't know the safety of the drug or medication, they may just recommend weaning. But, if you must wean quickly, prepare for some discomfort for both you and your baby. Sudden weaning may cause your breasts to become very full and uncomfortable. Expressing a small amount of milk may relieve the pressure. Don't remove too much milk, though, or you'll make more milk to replace it! The most uncomfortable portion of sudden weaning occurs in the first few days. Wearing a close-fitting bra that gives gentle, even pressure (such as a sports bra) may feel good. Ask your healthcare provider about whether a nonsteroidal anti-inflammatory drug like ibuprofen would be OK to take. This may make you more comfortable.

Your baby may be very upset by sudden weaning. She will still need lots of cuddles and snuggles from you. It may be difficult for her to be close to your breasts because she can smell your milk, which reminds her of nursing. Hold her with her back against your chest, and rock her. Make sure she has lots of opportunities to suckle on a bottle or pacifier to meet her comfort needs as well as her food needs.

The Breastfeeding Experience

PART FOUR

Lifestyle and Breastfeeding

How can I combine breastfeeding with
work or school?

Is it OK to exercise while breastfeeding?

What's a healthy diet for breastfeeding?

More ...

50. I don't want my baby to be too dependent on me. How can I prevent that from happening and keep breastfeeding?

All babies love their parents and want to be with them. Throughout your pregnancy your baby heard the sound of your heartbeat, voice, and breathing. It's not surprising that newborn babies feel most comfortable when these familiar sounds are within range. Newborns also have the amazing ability to identify the smell of their own mother from 2 hours after birth. It seems that the taste of each mother's amniotic fluid is similar to the scent of her body and her milk. So it's normal for your baby to want to be near you. Skin-to-skin contact is the best way to comfort and relax your baby.

Many mothers worry that they're making their babies dependent by giving in to their babies' need for contact. Human babies depend on their parents for survival. They're not able to fend for themselves in the world for many years. Giving your baby as much contact as he needs is the appropriate response. As your baby grows, he will become more interested in playing with his father, his brothers and sisters, and other family members. The time will come when those other people will be important to your baby.

Your partner, family members, and friends may not appreciate this. Some may feel envious of the special bond you have with your baby. Others may feel left out. It's a good idea to help other key support people find a special way to connect with the baby and support you and the baby.

Skin-to-skin contact is the best way to comfort and relax your baby.

In many cultures the mother's support circle steps in to take over the child care, cooking, cleaning, laundry, shopping, and other necessary household jobs and family responsibilities. This allows the mother to recover from birth and learn about the needs of the new baby. Unfortunately, such support does not exist for many modern mothers who may live hundreds of miles from their family and friends.

If you do have friends and family members who support you, it's a good idea to prepare a wish list for them. What kinds of household chores would you like help with? Would you like someone to pick up your dirty laundry and return it clean? Would you like to have frozen meals delivered? What foods does your family like to eat? Would it be helpful for someone to come clean the house or take your older children to the playground so you can take a nap with the baby? If you have a prepared list, it may be easier to respond when someone says, "Let me know if I can do anything for you."

51. I have older children. How can I keep them happy while I breastfeed the new baby?

Once you and your baby have mastered breastfeeding, nursings can be a great time to spend with your older children. You may read a special book to your children while you're nursing (because nursing requires only one arm to hold the baby, you can hold a book with the other one!). Other mothers tell stories or watch special videos with their children during feeding times. Some families keep a basket of special toys that come out only during feedings—this helps older children look forward to feeding times.

If an older child is jealous of the new baby, nursing in a sling helps distract the child's attention from the baby. While nursing in a sling, you can move about, even going for a walk or pushing the older child on a swing.

What if my older child asks to breastfeed?

When your child sees her new sibling nursing, it's only natural for her to want to have the same close relationship with you. Many mothers do breastfeed both a newborn and an older child, particularly when they have nursed the older child throughout pregnancy. This is called "tandem nursing." How would you feel about nursing two children? For some mothers, it's a helpful way to meet the needs of both children. For others, it's just too much. You are the only one who can determine what you would be comfortable with.

We recommend that you think about how you would feel about tandem nursing before your older child asks you about breastfeeding. Suppose that you have decided not to tandem-nurse. When your older child asks you about breastfeeding, you may want to respond by saying, "Breastfeeding is for babies. Would you like some special snuggle time with Mommy? Or would you like a special snack right now?"

On the other hand, if you've decided that you'd be interested in tandem nursing, you can respond positively to the request to breastfeed. Know that many children may have forgotten how to remove milk from the breast. So some children will try to suckle and then give up after a few attempts. You can find more guidance about tandem nursing in Question 73.

52. What can I do about people who aren't supportive of me breastfeeding?

It's truly unfortunate that some folks don't support your decision to breastfeed. You're making the healthiest choice for your baby and yourself—key people in your life should respect that, even if they're not comfortable with the thought of breastfeeding.

There are different ways to cope with a lack of support. One is to ignore it and go forward with breastfeeding. You can just say, "I'm sorry you don't support me. I'd prefer if you keep your doubts or feelings to yourself." You can agree to disagree with these folks. Or you can work to educate them about your viewpoint.

Alternatively, you could bring the people who don't support you to a breastfeeding counselor and ask her or him to speak to your support persons' concerns.

53. How can I combine breastfeeding with work or school?

Many, many mothers are successfully combining breastfeeding with work or school. It's best to speak with your employer or your school's health department during your pregnancy. Find out what kind of leave you can take after your pregnancy and how your work or school can accommodate your needs for some break time to express milk. It may be easier to advocate for yourself when you're pregnant than it is after the birth of your baby.

After you return to work or school, breastfeeding is a great way to stay connected with your baby. The hor-

mones associated with breastfeeding help you relax
after a busy day, and the automatic snuggling of breastfeeding is soothing to both of you. If your baby will be
in a day care setting with other children, continuing to
breastfeed can help your baby deal with the new germs
he will encounter.

There are several ways to combine breastfeeding and
separation from your baby for work or school. Some
women are able to take advantage of on-site child care.
These women may visit their babies during break periods to breastfeed. Other women have a day care
provider near their work, and someone brings the baby
to them or they go to the baby during lunch for a feeding. Others express breast milk to be fed to the baby
the next day either while they're at work or school or
while they're at home. Some women collect lots of milk
during their maternity leave and freeze it in small
amounts. Yet other women choose not to express their
milk but provide formula for the day care provider to
feed the baby and continue to breastfeed when they're
with the baby.

How can I express milk at work or school?

Most women who will be separated from their baby for
8 hours or more per day find that it takes them three
15- to 20-minute segments throughout a day (45 minutes to an hour total) to collect enough milk for the
baby to receive the next day. For working women, this
may happen during a morning break, lunch break, and
afternoon break. For those at school, milk may be expressed between classes or during lunch.

Lifestyle and Breastfeeding

Where can I go to express milk?

The bathroom is not the best possible location. If you have a desk job, you may be able to express milk while you're working at your desk. If not, is there an office or room with a door that you could use for pumping? It would be nice to have some privacy so you don't have to worry about someone walking in on you. If you're at school, the nurse's office or infirmary should be able to find a space for pumping. You will want to think about where you will store expressed milk. Many women use a small lunch-size cooler with a refreezable ice pack to store bottles of milk.

If you cannot find a way to express milk at work or school, you can still successfully breastfeed. You might want to consider a pump that can be worn at work under your clothing and operated without others knowing (such as the WhisperWear™ pump). When your baby is older and your milk supply is established, you may be successful with breastfeeding when you are home, and expressing only once during work hours. You can find information about other methods of expressing milk in Questions 39 and 40.

How much milk will I need to express for my baby?

The amount of milk your baby will take depends on his age and appetite. If you're expressing for a young baby, it's best to package the milk in 1- or 2-ounce amounts. Why? Because young babies often don't take more than a few ounces per feeding. Any leftover milk at the end of the feeding should be discarded. So you don't want 3 ounces of a 4-ounce bottle discarded! See Questions 39 and 41 for more information about expressing, storing, and feeding human milk.

For babies older than 6 months of age, solid foods—such as fruits, vegetables, cereals, yogurt, meats, and other foods—may provide additional calories. You may not need to leave as much milk for your baby after the age of 6 months. You'll want to make sure that containers of your milk are clearly labeled, in permanent marker, with your baby's name. You may also want to put a sticker with the date expressed on each container so that old milk can be identified and discarded if not used. Make sure that your child care provider knows how to handle your milk safely. The US Department of Agriculture has a helpful series of pamphlets for parents and day care providers on safe storage and handling of your milk (see the Appendix).

54. Is it OK to exercise while breastfeeding?

Absolutely. Exercise has many benefits. Ask your obstetric care provider for approval before starting a postpartum exercise program. When you begin exercising, start gradually. Walking is a great exercise that you can enjoy with your baby. Some women enjoy mom-and-baby yoga, belly dancing, or exercise classes. Others like to jog, swim, dance, or go to the gym. Choose an activity that you enjoy because it will be easier to continue with than one you find boring or difficult.

Ask your obstetric care provider for approval before starting a postpartum exercise program.

You may have heard that your baby may not like the taste of your milk after exercise. When people exercise strenuously, **lactic acid** can build up temporarily in the bloodstream. Some people have wondered whether lactic acid in the blood finds its way into breast milk and bothers the baby. Studies have examined the effects of exercise on lactic acid in milk, finding that only maxi-

Lactic acid
the breakdown product of energy stored in the muscles that is released during intense exercise, such as sprinting

mal exercise, such as marathon running, increases lactic acid levels in milk. There's no evidence of lactic acid in the milk of women who exercise moderately. Even if lactic acid is present in milk, it's there for a short time and may not be noticed by the baby.

Do make sure that you have a comfortable bra to exercise in. During the early weeks of breastfeeding, you may need a larger bra or sports bra for comfort. Make sure your bra does not pinch or squeeze your breasts because that can decrease milk flow.

Exercise can really help you gain strength and increase your ability to cope well with the demands of mothering.

55. What's a healthy diet for breastfeeding?

Eating well is always important. When we eat well, our bodies function at their peak. After pregnancy and childbirth, your body needs to rebuild its store of many nutrients, so a healthy diet is a great idea. An example of a healthy diet for women is in Table 10. Any healthy diet will be healthy for breastfeeding. Healthy diets include lots of fruits, vegetables, whole-grain foods, lean protein sources, and water.

It's best to vary the foods you eat. Variety provides a wide range of nutrients, vitamins, and minerals to keep your body strong and healthy and to give you lots of energy. Your nursing baby is also exposed to the flavors of the foods you eat when you're nursing. Studies suggest that babies are more likely to accept as toddlers those foods that their mothers consumed during pregnancy and lactation. Why? Researchers think the flavors of the solid foods are not new to breastfed babies—they tasted those

Table 10   A Healthy Diet for Postpartum Women

- At least five to nine servings of fruits and vegetables daily. Brightly colored vegetables and fruits are particularly healthful, especially those that are dark and leafy (spinach, kale, etc.), deep orange (cantaloupes, sweet potatoes, etc.), and dark red/blue (beets, blueberries, etc.). Fruit juice should be consumed in small amounts (4–8 ounces) and be 100% juice. It's best to have only one serving of your daily fruits from juice. The rest should be from fresh or frozen unsweetened fruits and vegetables. Try to eat more vegetables than fruit because they're richer in overall nutrients.

- Four to six or more servings of healthy grain foods. A serving of grain foods is a 1-ounce slice of bread, a half cup of cooked grains, or five to seven crackers. At least half of your grain-food choices should come from whole grains (100% whole-wheat breads and pastas, corn or whole-wheat tortillas, regular or old-fashioned oats, brown rice, whole-grain crackers, etc.).

- At least two servings of lean protein foods daily, such as beans (pinto, kidney, garbanzo, etc.—not string beans); tofu; nuts (including butters made from peanuts and other nuts) and seeds; fish; lean cuts of chicken, turkey, beef, pork, and other lean meats; and eggs. A serving size is 2–3 ounces of cooked meat, 1 cup of cooked beans, two eggs, or 4 tablespoons of nuts or seeds.

- Two to three servings of calcium-rich foods, such as low-fat or fat-free milk, yogurt, cheese, or calcium-fortified soy or rice milk. A serving is 1 cup of milk or yogurt, or 1.5–2 ounces of cheese.

- Two tablespoons of healthy fats daily. Healthy fats include mono- and polyunsaturated, unhydrogenated fats—such as olive and canola oils; margarines based on those oils; avocados; nuts; and seeds. Avoid excess saturated fats found in butter, hydrogenated oils (those that are solid at room temperature), trans fats, full-fat dairy products, and foods fried in oil.

- Some foods contribute extra nutrients. For example, 1 cup of yogurt can be counted as both a calcium serving and a protein serving. A cup of cooked beans is both a protein serving and a vegetable serving.

flavors in their mother's milk and amniotic fluid. So eating well may not just help you feel well; it may also decrease the chances that your baby will be a picky eater!

Aren't there foods I should avoid?

You have probably heard that there are foods you can't eat when breastfeeding. For example, the gassy foods you eat will give your baby gas. This is not true for the vast majority of babies. There are no foods that nursing mothers should avoid. There are, however, many foods that nursing mothers should eat only occasionally and in small amounts because they're too rich in calories, not because they will trouble most babies. This category includes such foods as rich desserts, baked goods, sweets, ice cream, soda, fried foods, butter, cream, chips, and other snack foods. If you're craving sweets, try to substitute fruits, vegetables, or healthy grain snacks. Snacking on apple slices dipped in peanut butter or carrot sticks dipped in yogurt mixed with lemon juice and dill may help replace the sweet, crunchy, or savory treats you crave.

I'm a vegetarian. How will that affect my baby?

A well-balanced vegetarian diet is a healthy diet. Vegetarian women, however, may encounter a few challenges after having a baby and during breastfeeding. One is getting enough iron to replace the iron they gave their baby during pregnancy. A good thing about breastfeeding for vegetarian women is that they lose less blood and begin menstruation later. That gives their body a chance to catch up. Blackstrap molasses, beans, dark leafy greens, whole grains, and dried figs and apricots are good sources of iron. Eating iron-rich foods in combination with vitamin C–rich foods (such as broccoli, greens, strawberries, citrus fruits, etc.) helps the body absorb more iron. If you're a vegetarian woman with postpartum **anemia**, ask your healthcare provider if you may need extra iron above the amount in your prenatal vitamin to rebuild your iron stores.

If you follow a vegan diet (which excludes all foods of animal origin, including milk products, honey, etc.), you will most likely need to take supplements for vitamin

Anemia

a condition in which the blood is deficient in red blood cells, in hemoglobin, or in total volume; typically refers to iron-deficiency anemia

B$_{12}$, iron, vitamin D, and **DHA** (**docosahexaenoic acid**, a long-chain polyunsaturated fat found in coldwater fish). Using iodized salt is a good idea for vegans, who may have difficulty getting enough iodine from their diets. Continue to eat a wide variety of foods during the time after birth to rebuild your body stores of other essential nutrients.

I'm not a vegetarian, but I don't drink milk. How will that affect my breast milk?

It's not necessary to drink milk to make milk. Our bodies use calcium from our diet and our body stores to provide calcium for our babies. Many women avoid milk and other dairy foods. Perhaps you don't like the taste of milk. Perhaps you are **lactose** intolerant, meaning that you cannot comfortably digest the sugar found in all liquid animal milks. (Please note that **lactose intolerance** is a problem only for older children and adults. It's extremely rare for a baby to be lactose intolerant. Most babies who have difficulty with cow's milk have an allergic reaction to the protein in that milk. Lactose is a sugar—allergies only happen in response to proteins.) Avoiding milk for either reason does not pose a problem for breastfeeding. Talk with your healthcare provider or nutritionist to make sure you're taking in enough calcium and vitamin D to meet your body's needs. Your milk will be just fine without drinking cow's milk, but your body may need a bit more calcium and vitamin D to keep your bones strong and your health excellent.

I had gastric bypass surgery before this pregnancy. Should I breastfeed?

Women can breastfeed after gastric bypass surgery. After your surgery, your body cannot as efficiently

Docosahexaenoic acid (DHA)

a long-chain polyunsaturated fatty acid believed to support an infant's rapidly developing nervous system

Lactose

a sugar found only in mammalian milk

Lactose intolerance

a condition occurring in some adults in which the body does not produce adequate amounts of lactase, causing abdominal bloating, gas, and pain when foods containing lactose are consumed

Lifestyle and Breastfeeding

absorb and digest food as it once could. So eating a wide variety of healthy foods is important to ensure that you get enough nutrients. Be sure to continue to take any vitamins and dietary supplements prescribed by your healthcare provider. Let your baby's healthcare provider know about your surgery so that he or she can determine your baby's need for vitamin supplements.

56. Is it OK to lose weight while breastfeeding?

Yes. In fact, making milk burns extra calories, so you should expect a gradual weight loss through the months after birth. Studies have found that breastfed babies continue to grow well while their mothers lose 1–2 pounds per week. As always, it's important to maintain a healthy diet to protect your body's nutrient stores. It's not a good idea to try to lose more than 2 pounds per week during this time because your body is trying to rebuild muscle and other tissue lost in the pregnancy.

It takes more than a year for a body to completely rebuild after childbirth. Continue to eat well even after you wean. Women have an opportunity to build stronger bones during the weaning period. Crash dieting during that time limits the recovery of bone and other tissue. Being pregnant and taking care of a new baby are hard work—you deserve a healthy diet during these crucial times!

57. Should I take special vitamins while breastfeeding?

If you eat a healthy, balanced diet, you may not need extra vitamins and minerals while you're breastfeeding. If you have certain medical conditions (e.g., anemia) or have had certain operations (e.g., gastric bypass surgery) or if you eat a very restricted diet, you should consult with your healthcare provider or nutritionist about your particular needs.

Many healthcare providers continue to prescribe prenatal vitamins for breastfeeding women. Ask your healthcare provider whether this is recommended for you.

58. Is it normal to be moody while breastfeeding?

Yes! After giving birth, many women experience mood swings. (Mood swings can start during pregnancy also.) The most common type of mood disturbance experienced is called the "baby blues." This is thought to affect more than 75% of new mothers, causing them to be unexpectedly weepy in the early days of their baby's life. Hormonal change may be linked to mood disturbances. Many other things that happen after birth contribute to moody behavior, such as sleep deprivation, adjusting to the parenting role, a lack of real support for new families, and the demanding schedule of life with a baby.

Women have different responses to these changes. Some become depressed. Others feel anxious and may have anxiety attacks. For some women, the experience of giving birth may have caused symptoms of posttraumatic stress disorder. Rarely, women can have psychotic episodes after birth. If any of these disorders sound familiar to you, don't be afraid. Having a mood disorder after giving birth is a medical problem. Ask for help. Don't let anyone tell you that your feelings are not acceptable or are just in your head.

Having a mood disorder after giving birth is a medical problem. Ask for help.

If you're feeling moody, it's important to talk about your feelings with someone you trust. Don't hold it all inside. If your partner, family members, and friends cannot help you with your feelings or if you become more moody, call your healthcare provider's office and ask to speak with the nurse. It's important to pay attention to your feelings.

You can use the Edinburgh Postnatal Depression Scale, a 10-question quiz, to track how you're feeling. (See Table 11.) You can also find resources online. Some are listed in the Appendix. Many communities now have new-mothers groups that focus on the emotional aspects of motherhood. Please reach out for help.

59. I just don't feel like having sex much. Is that normal for breastfeeding women?

Yes. After giving birth, many women cannot imagine wanting to make love right away or ever having another baby. These feelings are likely to change with time. Regardless of how you choose to feed your baby, you're likely to experience a change in how you feel about sex in the time after birth.

How you feel about making love after giving birth can be influenced by many things, including:

- Hormones. Key hormones that influence sexual desire change drastically immediately after delivery. While you're breastfeeding, these hormones are present in different levels, causing changes such as dryness of the vagina, milk flow on stimulation of the nipples, etc.
- Fatigue. It's hard to be interested in sex when you're exhausted from getting up at night to feed your baby.

Table 11   Edinburgh Postnatal Depression Scale

Edinburgh Postnatal Depression Scale (EPDS)

The EPDS was developed for screening postpartum women in outpatient, home visiting settings, or at the 6–8 week postpartum examination. It has been utilized among numerous populations including U.S. women and Spanish speaking women in other countries. The EPDS consists of 10 questions. The test can usually be completed in less than 5 minutes. Responses are scored 0, 1, 2, or 3 according to increased severity of the symptom. Items marked with an asterisk (*) are reverse scored (i.e., 3, 2, 1, and 0). The total score is determined by adding together the scores for each of the 10 items. Validation studies have utilized various threshold scores in determining which women were positive and in need of referral. Cut-off scores ranged from 9 to 13 points.

Therefore, to err on safety's side, a woman scoring 9 or more points or indicating any suicidal ideation—that is she scores 1 or higher on question #10—should be referred immediately for follow-up. Even if a woman scores less than 9, if the clinician feels the client is suffering from depression, an appropriate referral should be made. The EPDS is only a screening tool. It does not diagnose depression—that is done by appropriately licensed health care personnel. Users may reproduce the scale without permission providing the copyright is respected by quoting the names of the authors, title and the source of the paper in all reproduced copies.

Instructions for Users

1. The mother is asked to underline 1 of 4 possible responses that comes the closest to how she has been feeling the previous 7 days.
2. All 10 items must be completed.
3. Care should be taken to avoid the possibility of the mother discussing her answers with others.
4. The mother should complete the scale herself, unless she has limited English or has difficulty with reading.

Name:

Date:

Address:

Baby's Age:

As you have recently had a baby, we would like to know how you are feeling. Please UNDERLINE the answer which comes closest to how you have felt IN THE PAST 7 DAYS, not just how you feel today.

(continues)

Table 11   Edinburgh Depression Scale   *(continued)*

Here is an example, already completed.

I have felt happy:

Yes, all the time

Yes, most of the time

No, not very often

No, not at all

This would mean: "I have felt happy most of the time" during the past week. Please complete the other questions in the same way.

In the past 7 days:

1. I have been able to laugh and see the funny side of things

As much as I always could

Not quite so much now

Definitely not so much now

Not at all

2. I have looked forward with enjoyment to things

As much as I ever did

Rather less than I used to

Definitely less than I used to

Hardly at all

*3. I have blamed myself unnecessarily when things went wrong

Yes, most of the time

Yes, some of the time

Not very often

No, never

4. I have been anxious or worried for no good reason

No, not at all

Hardly ever

Yes, sometimes

Yes, very often

*5. I have felt scared or panicky for no very good reason

Yes, quite a lot

Yes, sometimes

No, not much

No, not at all

*6. Things have been getting on top of me

Yes, most of the time I haven't been able to cope at all

Yes, sometimes I haven't been coping as well as usual

No, most of the time I have coped quite well

No, have been coping as well as ever

*7. I have been so unhappy that I have had difficulty sleeping

Yes, most of the time

Yes, sometimes

Not very often

No, not at all

*8. I have felt sad or miserable

Yes, most of the time

Yes, quite often

Not very often

No, not at all

*9. I have been so unhappy that I have been crying

Yes, most of the time

Yes, quite often

Only occasionally

No, never

*10. The thought of harming myself has occurred to me

Yes, quite often

Sometimes

Hardly ever

Never

Source: Cox, J. L., Holden, J. M., & Sagovsky R. (1987). Edinburgh postnatal depression scale (EPDS). *British Journal of Psychiatry 150,* 782–786.

- Body image. It takes a while for our bodies to recover their normal shape and appearance after pregnancy. How you and your partner feel about these changes can affect your sexual confidence.
- Physical discomfort. Birth experiences—such as an episiotomy, cesarean delivery, or tailbone (coccyx) injury—can cause lingering pain in the genital area. Seek help from your healthcare provider for any continuing pain.

Remember that your partner (if you have one) experiences many of these same changes with you. Keep the lines of communication open by talking about your feelings and concerns about your sex drive. Make your partner aware of how much you appreciate the support, love, and care that are provided. Make time for nonsexual cuddling and snuggling. Partners need love, too! Many feel a little envious of the baby who is so physically close to you. Try to imagine how you would feel if your partner were nursing your baby.

60. I have a cold (or the flu). What can I take?

While you're breastfeeding, it's important to check the safety of any medication you're thinking of taking. This includes prescription drugs, as well as those you can purchase over the counter, including cold remedies, herbs, vitamins, minerals, and other dietary supplements. Don't assume that something is safe because it's available without a prescription. And don't think that a natural product is safer—it may not be! The safety of a drug during breastfeeding cannot be predicted from its safety during pregnancy. This means that drugs or supplements your doctor said were OK during pregnancy may not be safe during breastfeeding.

Always check drugs out with your healthcare provider, but know that the resources available to him or her may not have specific information about the safety of many drugs during breastfeeding. If you have access to the Internet, you can check out drugs in the National Library of Medicine's LactMed search engine (see the Appendix). Your breastfeeding support person may have access to other resources, such as the reference *Medications and Mother's Milk* (also in the Appendix). Perhaps you're asking about cold and flu medication because you're experiencing symptoms of mastitis. Mastitis is an inflammation of the breast, which involves feelings of swelling, warmth, redness, and discomfort in the breast. As mastitis gets worse, many mothers begin to feel overall aching and fatigue. Take a look at your breasts in the mirror if you have these symptoms, and look for swollen, red, sore areas. See Question 43 for more information about mastitis. You can continue to breastfeed with this condition, but you will want to contact your healthcare provider to discuss how to resolve it.

If I have just a cold or the flu, should I keep breastfeeding my baby?

Yes. Continuing to breastfeed will help protect your baby against the germs that have caused your cold or flu. These germs are in your home, and your baby has been exposed to them. You're making antibodies to these germs, and your antibodies, which are present in your milk, will help your baby fight the germs. It's always important to practice careful hand washing, but no time is more important than when you're ill. Wash your hands well every time you blow your nose. Wash your hands before picking up your baby and before touching your nipple area.

What if I'm sick with something else?

There are very few illnesses that require mothers to be separated from their babies. If you're diagnosed with tuberculosis, you may not be in proximity of your baby until you have received antituberculosis medication for 2 weeks or so. A few illnesses that cause eruptions on the nipple area are dangerous for breastfeeding babies. These include herpes and chicken pox lesions on the mother's breast in an area where the baby's mouth contacts the skin.

See Table 1 for a list of other conditions that may require a woman to stop breastfeeding.

Lifestyle and Breastfeeding

61. Can I get a perm, color my hair, whiten my teeth, or get a tattoo while breastfeeding?

Treatments for your hair and your teeth are compatible with breastfeeding. The chemicals used are absorbed into your body at very low rates; thus, they're not a problem for babies.

Tattooing with dirty needles could expose you to hepatitis or other infections. Because of this risk, tattooing is not recommended during either pregnancy or breastfeeding.

62. I'm planning to travel. How can I integrate travel plans with breastfeeding?

Breastfeeding can be very compatible with travel. Traveling can be easier with a breastfed baby than with a formula-fed baby. You don't have to worry about refrigerating formula and cleaning bottles. And even in hot climates, your baby will not need extra water (your milk is an excellent source of water for your baby). Continue to pay attention to your baby's feeding cues, and feed frequently during your travels (it's easier to miss cues when you're busy).

If you're concerned about breastfeeding in public during your travels, you may want to bring along a soft fabric baby sling. When you're "wearing" your baby in a sling, those around you will be less aware that you're nursing. Choosing loose tops with an overshirt or shawl can further disguise your breastfeeding.

Traveling without Your Breastfeeding Baby

Managing your milk supply while traveling away from your breastfeeding baby takes some planning. However, many women travel successfully, whether for a few days or for several weeks.

Weeks before you travel, decide how your baby will be fed during your absence. If you want to provide enough milk for your baby during a separation of more than a day, you will want to begin to collect your milk. (See Questions 39 and 41 for tips about collecting and storing milk.) Freeze your milk so that it will be usable for many months.

The next decision is whether you wish to continue to maintain your milk supply during your travels with the goal of resuming breastfeeding on your return. If this is your plan, you will want to learn hand expression or bring along a sturdy breast pump. If you will be traveling abroad, check into appropriate voltage and plug adapters for your destinations. Other supplies to consider are milk containers. If you plan to carry or ship milk back to your baby, you will need multiple storage containers. For long trips, you may want to consider single-use plastic collection bags that may be purchased from some breast pump companies. Using regular food storage bags for storing human milk is not recommended.

If you will be parted from your baby for only a few days, consider a portable cooler with refreezable ice packs. If you will not have access to refrigeration and ice, it may not be safe to save the expressed milk. However, continuing to express your milk will keep your

Weeks before you travel, decide how your baby will be fed during your absence.

Lifestyle and Breastfeeding

133

body making milk so that you can resume breastfeeding when you're reunited with your baby.

Current air travel regulations require that you report any human milk that you hand-carry onto an airplane. Check the Transport Security Administration Web site (www.tsa.gov) for specific regulations regarding gel packs and breast milk in containers on airplanes within the United States or those that take-off or land in the United States. Safety requirements may be different for other countries. The Centers for Disease Control and Prevention can provide guidance about immunizations needed for travel and other considerations.

Many women who are apart from their babies experience periods of sadness. Many babies also experience distress when separated from their mothers. When reunited with their mothers, even after only a few hours' separation, babies react in different ways. Some are overjoyed to see their mothers and want to nurse right away. Others may hold back, acting hurt or indifferent, and may refuse to breastfeed. In this situation offering your breast to a sleepy or sleeping baby may be an easy way to restart your breastfeeding relationship with him.

PART FIVE

You and Your Family

Does breastfeeding affect my
menstrual periods and my fertility?

My baby was fine with breastfeeding but now seems
easily distracted. How can I make him breastfeed?

When should I wean my baby?
How does weaning work?

More...

63. Does breastfeeding affect my menstrual periods and my fertility?

The vaginal bleeding women experience postpartum is called **lochia**. The bleeding may appear similar to a period, but you should not use tampons, only pads. The bleeding is expected to change colors. (See Table 12.) If the red discharge continues beyond the first few days, call your healthcare provider. Continuing to have a red discharge could indicate that your body has retained placental fragments. These could impact your milk supply because the hormones that continue to make mature milk are based on the complete delivery of the placenta.

Lochia
the discharge from the uterus after birth

If you don't have the changes in color listed in Table 12 or if your discharge is heavy (more than a pad every 2 hours) or clumpy, be sure to call your healthcare provider.

Some women find that their period is delayed for a time after birth when breastfeeding. Not all women experience this delay. When your period returns (and possibly before your period returns), you may ovulate and could get pregnant. Do not count on a lack of menses to mean that you're not ovulating.

If you're trying to get pregnant again, you may think you need to wean from breastfeeding. This is seldom the case. If you're going through in vitro fertilization

Table 12   Postpartum Vaginal Discharge

- In the first few days postpartum: a red-colored uterine discharge
- After the first few days: brownish, paler, more clear-colored discharge
- Second and 3rd week postpartum: thicker, yellowish discharge
- By the 5th week: healing should be nearly complete or complete as evidenced by absence of discharge

(IVF) methods, your healthcare providers may ask you to wean because of the medications that are often used with IVF. For most families who are trying to conceive without medical intervention, weaning is not necessary.

64. Can I count on breastfeeding for birth control if I'm trying not to get pregnant? If I'm trying to get pregnant, will breastfeeding interfere?

You may think that you cannot get pregnant when breastfeeding. You can. Or you may worry that to have another baby, you will need to wean. You usually don't. Breastfeeding (with very specific guidelines; see the Lactational Amenorrhea Method [LAM] in Figure 24) may provide birth control for the first 6 months. If you don't meet one or more of the specific LAM guidelines, you'll need another method of birth control to avoid a pregnancy. After 6 months of breastfeeding, LAM is no longer an effective strategy.

65. What birth control methods are safe and effective during breastfeeding?

All barrier methods—including cervical caps, condoms, diaphragms, foam, etc.—are acceptable for nursing mothers. Most nursing mothers have vaginal dryness and are more comfortable when additional lubrication is used.

Among the hormonal methods, progestin-only forms of birth control are options for nursing mothers after the early weeks (usually after 6 weeks, when breastfeeding is well established). These include birth control pills and the injectable drug Depo-Provera. Progestin-

The Lactational Amenorrhea Method (LAM) is presented as an algorithm, below.

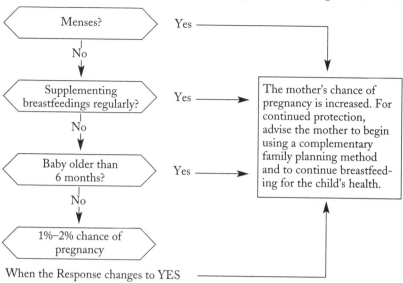

Figure 24   The Lactational Amenorrhea Method. Source: Adapted from Labbok, M., Cooney, K., & Coly, S. (1994). *Guidelines: Breastfeeding, family planning, and the Lactation Amenorrhea Method—LAM.* Washington, DC: Institute for Reproductive Health.

only birth control options are considered to impact milk supply less than estrogen-and-progestin combination birth control options. The hormones from a progestin-only birth control product can still impact your milk supply, especially if they're started before the baby is 6 weeks old. For this reason, an advantage of progestin-only birth control pills, over injectable birth control, is that if you notice a decrease in your milk supply, you can stop taking the pills and work to increase your milk supply again.

The Lactational Amenorrhea Method is another option (see Figure 24). Research studies indicate that the cumulative pregnancy rate using LAM is 0.9–1.2%, similar to other types of birth control.

66. I'm pregnant but still nursing my first child. Should I stop breastfeeding? Could nursing cause me to have a miscarriage?

An increased risk of miscarriage because of nursing during pregnancy has never been documented. Of course, if you have a history of miscarriage, you may not want to do anything, such as breastfeeding or having sex, that will stimulate oxytocin. This is because oxytocin is released during sex and while breastfeeding, and is also the hormone that contracts the uterus during labor.

At some point during the pregnancy, your breast milk will revert back to colostrum, probably by around 5 months. This may be an issue for the nursing baby. Colostrum is packed with antibodies and nutrients, so it's still protective and nutritious. But if the baby is less than a year old, his total food intake needs to be evaluated. If the nursing baby is a toddler, colostrum may cause loose stools (colostrum is a laxative). If your toddler is potty-training, this laxative effect may be a problem!

67. My in-laws say formula was good enough for my husband, and he turned out OK. What do I say to them?

Mothers 20, 30, or 40 years ago made the best decisions they could based on the information that was known then. Tell your in-laws that you know that they made the best decision they could with the information that was available and that you're making the best decision today. Over the past 30 years, tremendous research on breastfeeding and formula has shown overwhelmingly the benefits of breastfeeding. That doesn't mean that mothers decades ago did anything wrong, but it also doesn't mean that mothers today need to follow the past without considering this new knowledge.

68. My family traditions involve supplementing babies with teas. Is this OK?

As you journey through parenthood, it's wonderful to think about which family traditions and cultural beliefs you will share with your new child. You may decide to celebrate certain holidays and choose dietary options that are part of your traditions. Whatever you choose to pass on, consider how your decisions will affect the baby.

If a baby is fed something other than breast milk—tea, for example—will she consume less of the highly nutritious breast milk? What is in the tea? Some herbs can cause problems with a baby, such as allergies. Is the tradition important because of a condition or situation that no longer exists? For example, babies used to be given water bottles because formula was too strong. Breastfed babies don't need water bottles—it's important not to apply outdated formula-feeding traditions to breastfeeding.

69. My baby was fine with breastfeeding but now seems easily distracted. How can I make him breastfeed?

When babies turn 4–6 months old, they become increasingly aware of the world around them. They may concentrate on toys or the environment. It's amazing to watch them learn and grow. These distractions can, however, make breastfeeding challenging—for example, if the baby becomes more interested in the person walking into the room or the button on your sweater than breastfeeding.

There are several techniques to try. Nursing in a quiet, dark room can sometimes help. So can cluster feeding (several feedings in a row) when the baby is interested. One mother would say to her 6-month-old, "OK, sweetie, it's time to nurse like a little baby." Breastfeeding when the baby is drowsy or semiawake may be a great chance to get another feeding in. When babies are distracted during the day, they sometimes make up for it at night and have more periods of wakefulness or exhibit more hunger cues. Cluster feeding in the evening hours may help. Sometimes several short feedings can even tank up the baby to sleep better at night.

Breastfeeding when the baby is drowsy or semiawake may be a great chance to get another feeding in.

70. How should I start solid foods?

Many national and international groups are changing their recommendations to say that babies should be exclusively breastfed for about 6 months and then started on solid foods while continuing to breastfeed. This is a change from the old recommendation, which was starting solid foods at 4 months. The extra months of maturity make a difference with how the feedings work and what foods to begin with.

Six-month-old babies shouldn't be spoon fed the way we used to feed younger babies. They have a pincer grasp and can pick up food with their fingers. They have tongue control and don't push food back out of their mouths the way younger babies do. You don't need to scrape food off their chin and refeed them.

Prior solid food recommendations were based on adding foods to complement homemade baby milk, not breast milk. Today nutritionists and pediatricians are thinking about the best first foods for breastfeeding babies. These are thought to be foods high in zinc and iron, such as meat. Foods that your baby can pick up, such as round dry cereals, are also good choices. When babies begin solid foods at 6 months, they progress to family foods fairly quickly. Your baby's doctor will be able to give you individualized recommendations for your baby.

71. When should I wean my baby? How does weaning work?

The recommendation from health and professional authorities is to nurse exclusively for 6 months, add solid foods around 6 months, and continue to breastfeed for 1 year—or 2, or 3, or more.

Research has shown that breastfeeding's health benefits increase in the second half of the 1st year. Breast milk continues to be nutritious, even increasing in calories and nutrients as time goes by. As long as both a mother and her baby enjoy nursing, they should continue to do so.

When the mother decides to wean, there are some strategies that seem to work best. First, think about the baby's nutrition. If the baby is less than a year old, she will need formula. If the baby is more than a year old, her nutrition is still a consideration. How will she get these nutrients? Cow's milk? Whole-milk yogurt?

With all babies, whether less than or more than a year old, their emotional needs are also part of the equation. Babies will still need the snuggling, loving, and holding that was part of the breastfeeding experience.

To start weaning, eliminate the baby's least favorite feeding first, and give the baby a substitution (expressed breastmilk or formula for those less than 1 year old; something else to eat or drink and a snuggle for babies older than 1 year). See how it goes the next day, continuing to substitute something for breastfeeding at that feeding time. After a couple of days (or whatever works for you), choose another feeding during the day to substitute for breastfeeding. Choosing one that isn't nap-time or bedtime is usually best in the beginning. Wean the baby from those feedings last.

If possible, slower weaning tends to be best. On occasion, mothers find themselves in a situation where they need to wean more quickly (e.g., for certain rare medical issues). If you need to wean more quickly, your breasts may become full and possibly engorged. Leaning into a dishpan with warm water can sometimes relieve this fullness. (See Figure 25.)

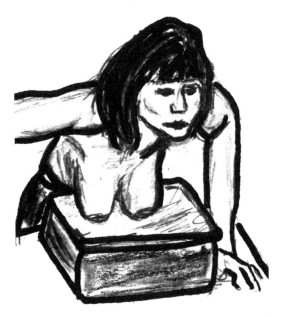

Figure 25 Soaking the Breasts
Lukewarm water (in this case, in a dishpan) helps relieve engorgement by encouraging the milk to flow.

72. I've heard that women can continue to nurse an older child as well as a new baby. Is that healthy?

Yes. Nursing two babies from different pregnancies (such as a toddler and a newborn) is referred to as "tandem nursing." It may be a relatively new phenomenon because previous generations thought that sex with pregnant women and nursing mothers was taboo. But well-nourished mothers can support breastfeeding while pregnant and go on to nurse two babies without ill effects.

73. I've just had a second baby and am nursing a toddler. Can you offer me some strategies to be sure that the baby gets enough milk?

Breastfeed the newborn first and frequently, and then breastfeed the older baby. The toddler will be able to eat other foods, so the baby must be the first priority even though the toddler may be more insistent! During the pregnancy and for the first days after the new baby is born, the toddler will receive colostrum, which is a laxative and could create looser stools for him.

Colostrum and breast milk have value and nutrition for both the baby and the toddler. The newborn baby should feed 10–12 times in 24 hours; babies more than a year old often nurse only in the morning, at bedtime, and sometimes before naps. The older baby should not be encouraged to nurse on a newborn schedule. Find other activities for the older baby, as described in Question 51.

The toddler may drive the milk supply, making the flow too fast for the newborn. If the baby is having difficulty with the abundance of milk (in other words, if the baby coughs at the breast or compresses the nipple to slow down the flow and creates sore nipples for you), try the Australian posture. With that position, you're "down under" the baby, and gravity works against the flow of the milk, causing it to slow down. (See Question 27.)

As with all babies, be sure your children go to pediatric appointments and weight checks to monitor their growth.

PART SIX

Breastfeeding Problems

My breasts hurt. What could be causing the pain?

I feel as if I'm not making enough milk.
What should I do?

My baby refuses to nurse on one breast.
What should I do?

More . . .

74. I have sore nipples and need help. What should I try?

If your nipples become sore or if breastfeeding is at all painful, it means that you need help. Breastfeeding should not be painful at all—not even for the first few seconds of the latch-on. If breastfeeding is at all uncomfortable or painful for you, you should ask a trained breastfeeding caregiver to observe a feeding and offer suggestions and techniques to improve the latch. In a research study conducted by the Healthy Children faculty, almost every case of sore nipples improved significantly when the latch was fixed. No mother had to give up on breastfeeding or feed her baby away from the breast when the latch was fixed. Review the feeding cues in Table 3 and the latching process described in Question 22.

Please don't try home remedies, such as creams, ointments, and salves. Anything you put on your nipple will go to your baby. Use solutions such as nipple shields only under the specific direction of your breastfeeding care provider because they can decrease the amount of milk your baby gets.

75. My breasts hurt. What could be causing the pain?

Because lactating breasts have a large blood supply, they bruise easily. There are a lot of nerves in the breasts as well, so pain there can be more painful than in other parts of the body. Please get help if you have any breast pain. Table 7 will help you with the symptoms of different types of breast problems.

76. My nipples don't stand out from my breast. How can I get my baby to latch on?

As the latch technique in Question 22 illustrates, the shape of the nipple is unimportant for latching.

Nipples that are inverted ("innies") before or during pregnancy will not necessarily stay inverted. The baby may be able to evert the nipple (see Figure 26). A breast pump may help pull the nipple out. And breasts and nipples can change through pregnancy, birth, and breastfeeding. So if your nipples appear flat (Figure 27) or inverted (Figure 28), they may not remain that way. (See Table 13 for the different grades of inverted nipples.)

You don't have to do anything during pregnancy to prepare your nipples. Prenatal nipple preparations (such as hard breast shells, exercises, or finger manipulation) aren't effective or recommended.

What is important is that nipples that are still inverted at the end of pregnancy are related to lower milk production and poorer weight gain for the baby. So if your nipples aren't out at the end of a nursing, please have an individualized assessment from a breastfeeding caregiver.

Table 13   Grades of Inverted Nipples

- Grade 1 inverted nipples are easily pulled out by suckling or a breast pump.
- Grade 2 inverted nipples are easily pulled out by suckling or a breast pump but don't maintain the projection once the baby's mouth leaves the nipple or the pump flange is removed.
- Grade 3 inverted nipples are difficult or impossible to pull out. Why? Perhaps because there are internal breast anomalies.

Source: Adapted from Han, S., & Hong, Y. G. (1999). The inverted nipple: Its grading and surgical correction. *Plastic Reconstructive Surgery, 104*(2), 389–395.

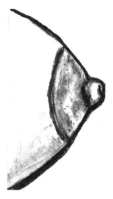

Figure 26 Everted Nipple
An everted nipple protrudes out from the areola.

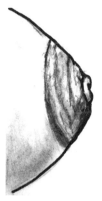

Figure 27 Flat Nipple
A flat nipple everts when it's cold or manually stimulated.

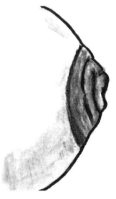

Figure 28 Inverted Nipple
An inverted nipple looks like a slit or a fold.

Here are some questions to consider and discuss with a breastfeeding caregiver:

- Does your nipple ever evert? If it usually does but now does not, could it be inverted because the breast is so full or engorged that the skin is tight?
- If the nipple doesn't evert (and was inverted prior to your baby's birth), does your nipple evert in response to cold or touch?
- Can your baby compress the areola (dark area around the nipple) and draw the nipple into his mouth, giving the nipple more form?

Other tips to keep in mind include the following:

- Some mothers find that using a hard plastic shell inside the bra in between feedings helps dry and evert the nipple.
- If you have inverted nipples, using a nipple shield may further reduce your milk supply and put the baby at increased risk for failure to thrive.
- Calorie-deprived babies act sleepy. The baby who sleeps more and acts content may not be getting enough milk. Frequent weight checks are the only way to know how the baby is doing with breastfeeding with an inverted nipple.

Sometimes nipples seem flat or inverted in the hours after the baby is born even if they never appeared this way before. It's possible that the medications and/or IV fluids you were given have temporarily affected your breasts and nipples. Even if your nipples are flat or inverted, you and your baby can still breastfeed. Spending time skin to skin can help. A good latch is also important. Sometimes babies make inverted nipples stick out (even if the nipples never have before) by latching on well.

If your nipples are flat or inverted after the first few days, be sure to ask for help. Some mothers choose to use hard breast shells in between breastfeedings to try to evert the nipple for the feeding. Some mothers find that pumping for a couple of minutes before feeding can help bring out a nipple. Please don't use a nipple shield unless you're working with a breastfeeding care-giver because it may decrease your milk transfer.

Even if your nipples are flat or inverted, you and your baby can still breastfeed.

It's very important to have frequent weight checks if you have inverted nipples, just to be certain that the baby is getting enough milk. There are many mothers who have inverted nipples and make plenty of milk, but there are also many mothers whose milk supply is com-promised because the baby isn't efficiently transferring milk. So it's important to be sure that you have enough milk and that the baby is able to transfer the milk, too.

77. My breasts are too full. How do I soften them and get the milk out?

Water works with lactation hormones to remove milk without telling your body to make a lot more milk. Getting in the shower or bathtub can help, but if you don't want to get wet all over, use a dishpan with warm water, as shown in Figure 25. Put the dishpan on a low table or coffee table. Lean your breasts into the dish-pan. Let the milk flow from your breasts. You may choose to gently massage your breasts. Be sure to be gentle with your breasts; don't bruise them or hurt them further.

Then nurse your baby. Nursing your baby frequently and effectively can help remove the pressure. You may wonder whether you should wear a bra. It's up to you and how the bra makes you feel. If the bra is too tight, it may cause more compression and may make your breasts hurt. If you don't wear a bra at all, your breasts may not feel comfortable because they probably feel heavier than usual. A correctly fitting bra or a tank top or camisole-style nursing bra may feel comfortable to you. Watch out for seams and underwires that could cause compression lines on the breast that may not be comfortable and can plug your ducts.

You may have been told that there are other solutions to engorgement or oversupply. One suggestion you might have heard involves putting cabbage on your breast. There is little evidence from research supporting this idea. You may wonder whether you should pump. Pumping may take the pressure off immediately, but the nipple stimulation and milk removal that comes from pumping will actually tell your body to make even more milk, which will make your breasts continue to feel overfull. If you have to pump, do so only for a couple of minutes, and try not to do it too often. Try the water technique described earlier.

What about warm compresses or ice packs with engorgement? There is no research showing that warm compresses or ice packs can help with engorgement, although either may make you fell more comfortable. Do what makes you feel best.

78. My breasts are really soft all of a sudden. Is something wrong?

Breasts change over the course of pregnancy, birth, and the early days of breastfeeding, and throughout lactation. If your breasts never changed during pregnancy, birth, or postpartum, be sure to tell your healthcare provider.

A few days after birth, your breasts will probably become very full. Then in the days following, one breast may get full while you're nursing on the other side. Your breasts may also get full between feedings. As you continue breastfeeding, your breasts get softer. This usually means that your breasts are getting used to lactating. If your baby has fewer stools or wet diapers in combination with your softer breasts, that is a concern, and you should bring this to the attention of the baby's doctor and your breastfeeding caregiver.

79. Breastfeeding seems to be taking a lot out of me. I'm having trouble getting out of bed. How do I know what's wrong with me?

If you're very tired postpartum, please bring this to the attention of your healthcare provider. Could it be related to anemia? Could it be related to childbirth blood loss? Is your thyroid working normally? Could you be depressed? Ask yourself the questions on the Edinburgh Postpartum Depression Scale (Table 11).

What is breastfeeding like for you? Is it comfortable? Does the baby nurse well and gain well? If breastfeeding sessions last more than 30 or 40 minutes long or the baby nurses more than 10–12 times in 24 hours, have a breatfeeding assessment with a skilled helper.

If I'm depressed, do I have to stop breastfeeding to take antidepressants?

No. There are many effective medications compatible with breastfeeding for your provider to choose from. Don't put off getting help because you think you're going to have to make a choice between feeling better and breastfeeding.

80. I feel as if I'm not making enough milk. What should I do?

If you're worried about your milk supply, an individualized breastfeeding assessment with before-and-after feeding weights using a digital scale accurate to 2 grams can help you estimate how much milk you're transferring. The specialized scale can tell you how much milk the baby took in at that feeding and estimate whether you're transferring enough milk for your baby's optimal growth.

You know that your baby is getting enough if:

- The baby has gained 1/2 ounce to 1 ounce a day after an initial loss of about 7% of body weight.
- The baby has regained her birth weight by about 10 to 14 days.
- The baby has 3 to 4 stools per day by days 3 to 5.
- The baby has 3 to 6 stools per day by days 5 to 7.

Less indicative of how the baby is doing with breastfeeding are urinations. Expect 3 to 5 urinations by days 3 to 5 and 4 to 6 urinations by days 5 to 7.

I have gone back to work, and I'm getting less milk when I pump. What should I do?

Here are some tips to build your milk supply:

- Check that the pump is working. Call the manufacturer if you suspect the pump may not be functioning properly. Even new, expensive pumps can malfunction, so it's worth checking them out.
- Check that you have all the pump parts.
- Determine whether your nipple moves freely when the pump is working. If your nipple is crushed in the flange tunnel, milk cannot flow. You may need a larger flange.
- If possible, when you're away from the baby, pump as often as the baby would feed.
- Nurse as often as you possibly can when you're with your baby.

81. My baby is not gaining enough weight. What should I do?

Expect newborns to gain about ½ ounce to 1 ounce per day. If your healthcare provider is concerned about your baby's weight gain, try the following:

Expect newborns to gain about ½ ounce to 1 ounce per day.

- Keep track of the number of times you feed your baby in a 24-hour period.
- Write down information about your baby's diapers (urinations and stools).
- Keep track of your baby's activities. Is your newborn baby sleeping for many hours without feeding? If so, keep the baby close to you and nurse on cue.
- Borrow or rent a baby weight scale with a breast milk intake function, if one is available in your community. A regular scale or a regular baby scale is

probably not accurate enough to measure breast milk intake.

- If your healthcare provider suggests supplementing, discuss the possibility of pumping and giving pumped milk to the baby as supplementation. If you're unable to pump enough for the baby, the baby still needs to eat enough, so formula or milk from a milk bank may be necessary. Perhaps you can feed the supplement with an at-breast feeder. That could help build up your milk supply while providing the baby with additional calories.

82. My baby cries a lot and may be gassy. Could something be wrong with my milk? Could it be something I'm eating?

Babies cry for many reasons. The baby may be hungry, tired, or in need of a diaper change. Or she may want to be held or snuggled. When you have tried all these things and the baby still cries, you may wonder what to do. Figuring out why the baby is crying or uncomfortable is very important.

Many babies have gastric discomfort. This does not necessarily indicate colic. Colic is defined by the "rule of 3": bouts of high-pitched crying lasting more than 3 hours per day, for more than 3 days per week, and for more than 3 weeks in a well-nourished, otherwise healthy baby. Mothers will often restrict their diet severely, often without positive effect on the baby's symptoms. If a dietary trial does not alleviate symptoms, you may want to ask your healthcare provider for suggestions for responding to your baby's discomfort. The baby may need to be examined to see whether she has a medical problem. Please see Question 93 about birth injuries.

A breastfed baby's crying is rarely related to the mother's diet. The one food that has been shown to relate to crying and colic is liquid cow's milk. Eliminating all liquid cow's milk from the mother's diet for 2 weeks should improve the baby's crying and colic, if that is the problem. If the baby's colic improves, the whey in her mother's diet may have been the cause. Many mothers find that steaming milk (such as used in a latte or cappuccino coffee) or cooking milk (such as in old-fashioned pudding and custard recipes) changes the milk protein enough so that it doesn't bother the baby. During the time the mother is eliminating cow's milk, she may benefit from consulting with a dietician.

There have been individual reports of other foods in the mother's diet causing reactions (e.g., eczema, proctocolitis) in the baby. Implicated foods include cow's milk, eggs, and fish—eaten singularly or in combination. There have also been reports of very rare cases in which a breastfed baby has symptoms of proctocolitis (blood in the stool). The situation is worrisome but not life threatening. It's an indication that the baby is sensitive to foods that the mother has eaten. Once the food is identified (either by removing foods from the mother's diet by trial and error or by testing the baby) and the baby no longer has blood in her stool, she should continue to be breastfed!

Spicy and gassy foods should only be excluded on a case-by-case basis, not as a general rule. Babies seem to like flavored milk best. In a research study, babies nursed almost twice as long when their mother had eaten garlic.

Breast milk conveys the flavors of the culture to the baby by flavoring the mother's milk. Babies seem to get used to the flavors in their mother's diet by swallowing amniotic fluid, which, like breast milk, takes on the flavors of the mother's food. Anthropologists and breastfeeding advocates believe that if you eat the flavors of your culture or family, your baby will recognize those flavors when she is old enough to start solid foods. The theory is that the child may be less likely to be a picky eater if she had breast milk that was flavored with the foods of your normal diet.

83. My baby refuses to nurse on one breast. What should I do?

It's OK for your baby to take only one breast at each feeding, but when the baby consistently refuses one breast, more evaluation is needed.

There are many possible reasons for a baby to refuse one side.

Reasons in newborns:

- The baby could be uncomfortable lying on that side (indicating possible bruising from birth or a birth injury). See Question 93.
- You may be holding the baby differently when nursing on that side. Is your hand or arm applying too much pressure on the back of the baby's head?
- Is your breast so full on that side that it's difficult for the baby to latch on to the breast?
- Is the baby so full from nursing on one side that the baby is refusing the other breast? Breastfeeding on one breast is fine if the baby is gaining well and has sufficient wet diapers and stools each day.
- Could the baby be congested or have an ear infection and be uncomfortable lying that way?
- Is there much more milk on that side?
- Is there less milk on that side?

If the baby has breastfed well in the past on that side and suddenly refuses that breast or if she refused that breast from birth, ask your healthcare provider whether an ultrasound of the breast would provide some insight into the baby's refusal. There's a rare but possible relationship between a baby's continued refusal to breastfeed on one breast and a cancer diagnosis in that breast even as many as 5 years after the baby refuses that breast.

Questions to consider with your baby's healthcare provider:

- Has the baby's weight gain, urinations and bowel movements been appropriate?
- Is there something different about how you hold the baby on one breast versus the other? What is the baby's body language when positioned on each breast?
- Does the baby always refuse the same breast (left or right)? Or is the baby refusing different breasts at different feedings?

Suggestions to encourage the baby to take the refused breast:

- Offer the baby the preferred breast first. When the baby releases that breast, move him to the other breast without shifting his body position. (See Figure 29.) If this position switch does not result in a latch on the less favored breast, then try other positions. (See Question 27.)
- If the baby prefers only one breast per feeding but does not always refuse the same breast, it's possible that he's receiving adequate milk at one breast and can't handle the volume from both breasts during a feeding. This is normal and means you have an abundant milk supply.

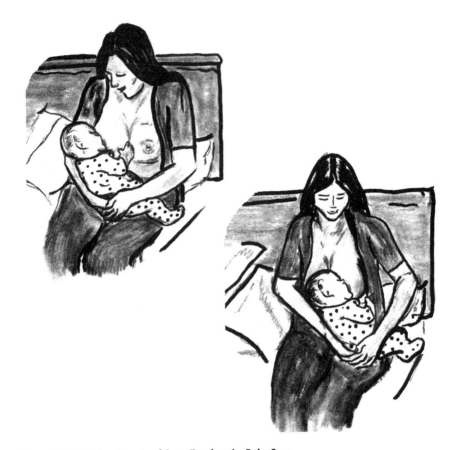

Figure 29 Switching Breasts without Turning the Baby Over
Nurse the baby on the second breast without turning the baby over.

- Differences in the rate of milk flow may also be the
  reason for one-sided feeding. It's common for each
  breast to have a different amount of milk and a different flow.

84. I've breastfed before, but this time it's harder. I have sore nipples, and my baby isn't happy. What's going on?

You may be experiencing a problem we call "oversupply." It almost seems as though once the breasts are
pros at making milk, they go overboard! Oversupply

rarely happens with first babies, although it may. Oversupply has the following characteristics:

- The baby gains rapidly, often a pound a week in the early weeks.
- The mother has sore nipples because the baby is clamping down on the nipple to slow the flow. If you've had a baby before (and especially if you breastfed previous babies), your body may be releasing the milk very fast. Your baby may be trying to slow down the flow by compressing the nipple (like a garden hose—if you put pressure on a garden hose, the water stops flowing).
- The baby isn't happy after feedings and often acts as if she wants another feeding. The baby spits up often and may have projectile vomiting.
- The baby has lots of large stools. The diaper usually can't hold the number of stools. Sometimes the stools are greenish rather than the expected yellow.

To deal with oversupply, you need to decrease the volume and flow of the milk. Try leaning back in the Australian or semireclined posture, where gravity works against the flow of the milk, slowing it down. (See Question 21.) If the baby has more control, you may no longer experience compression and pain. Once the baby takes less milk because he has more control, the remaining milk in your breast should signal your milk-making cells to begin making less milk.

To deal with oversupply, you need to decrease the volume and flow of the milk.

85. My baby's stools don't look normal. Is there something wrong?

Not necessarily. Babies' stools are not the same from day to day. They change in color (from black to yellow) and consistency:

Meconium

the first stool of a
newborn, varying
from greenish black
to light brown with a
tarry consistency

- Black or tar-colored stools. Stools in the first couple of days of life are called **meconium**. Expect them to be black or tarlike. Meconium stools are sticky. If the stools are black beyond the first couple of days of life, be sure to call your healthcare provider immediately.

- Greenish-brown stools. Transitional stools are greenish-brown and occur after the first couple of days of the baby's life. They're a mix of the blackish meconium stools and the typical yellow stools of breastfed babies. If your exclusively breastfed baby continues to have greenish-brown stools beyond the 4th day, call your pediatric care provider.

- Gray stools. Dull gray stools can indicate a metabolism problem. Please bring this to the attention of the baby's care provider.

- Bright-green stools. This could be a sign of oversupply (see Question 84) or poor latch (see Question 22).

- Watery yellow stools. This is what diarrhea looks like in breastfeeding babies. If the baby has watery yellow stools that do not have what looks like seeds or curds, then it could be diarrhea. Call your baby's healthcare provider.

- Seedy yellow stools. If the stools appear loose and yellow and have what looks like little seeds in it, they're typical breastfed baby stools.

- Harder, more formed brown stools. These stools indicate that the baby is receiving formula and foods other than breast milk. If that's not the case, discuss the baby's stools with your baby's healthcare provider.

- Bloody stools. Proctocolitis (or blood in the stools) can happen even with exclusively breastfed babies. Cow's milk formula or cow's milk in the mother's diet (although corn, soy, and chocolate have also been implicated) is thought to be the cause. In research studies the problem resolved within a week of removing the offending food from the mother's diet. If the baby is being fed the food directly (formula or solid food) the food is eliminated from the baby's diet.

- Red crystals in the diaper with the urine. This is often referred to as "brick dust urine." Let your healthcare provider know right away that your baby is having some red dust in her urine.

86. My baby has jaundice. What do I do?

A newborn baby who is diagnosed with jaundice probably has one of three different kinds of jaundice. If your baby has jaundice, ask which type of jaundice it is:

- Physiologic jaundice. The baby's body naturally eliminates **bilirubin** in the meconium stools. If the baby's immature body is having difficulty eliminating the bilirubin fast enough, the bilirubin builds up. That's called "hyperbilirubinemia." This happens in the early days postpartum, sometimes in the hospital and sometimes in the days after discharge.

Bilirubin

a by-product of the breakdown of the hemoglobin portion of red blood cells

- Pathologic jaundice. *Pathologic* means that there is some kind of disease or condition. Pathologic jaundice is often caused by newborn blood incompatibilities with the mother's blood (Rh and ABO) or liver disease.
- So-called breast milk jaundice. This is very rare. The theory is that something in the mother's milk interferes with the elimination of bilirubin. Another theory is that the baby lacks a particular liver enzyme. This type of jaundice happens after day 10.

Breastfeeding Suggestions for Babies with Physiologic Jaundice

- Babies with jaundice may be somewhat lethargic and sleepy. It's important to nurse often to help the baby stool (which will help the bilirubin get out of the baby's body).
- Milk expression and alternate massage during feedings may help increase the milk supply and intake.
- Sometimes breastfed babies with jaundice need supplementation to move the stools. Giving the baby expressed breast milk is best because colostrum is a laxative. If the baby is too sleepy and not nursing well, his nursing may not tell the mother's body to make enough milk. Pumping or hand expressing helps keep up the milk supply by raising the lactation hormones through nipple stimulation and milk removal. The pumped milk may be given to the baby or stored in the freezer for future feedings.

Breastfeeding Suggestions for Babies with Pathologic Jaundice

The onset of this type of jaundice has nothing to do with feeding, but because bilirubin is largely eliminated through the stools, breastfeeding and colostrum can help speed the process of removing bilirubin from the baby's body.

Breastfeeding Suggestions for Babies with So-Called Breast Milk Jaundice

This late-onset jaundice usually requires women to discontinue breastfeeding for 24 hours. During that 24-hour period, the baby is fed formula (not pumped milk). The baby's bilirubin levels should go down when he receives only formula because it doesn't have any species-specific ingredients. If the levels come down, then the jaundice is considered "late-onset jaundice," and the mother can resume breastfeeding.

If the bilirubin levels don't come down, the mother still resumes breastfeeding, and the baby will probably have additional lab work and tests to rule out other reasons for high bilirubin levels that are not related to the human elements in breast milk.

If your baby has breast milk jaundice, you should express your milk during the 24 hours of not breastfeeding to keep up your milk supply. Freeze that milk for later. Usually, a mother who has a baby with late-onset jaundice will find that subsequent babies may also have late-onset jaundice. The mothers and babies can go on to have a wonderful breastfeeding experience once the 24-hour test is over. Simply looking at the baby's coloring (because jaundice makes babies' skin look a bit orange or apricot) will not determine whether the levels have come down; lab work must be conducted. A healthcare provider may also order other medical interventions (such as special lights).

87. I've had breast surgery. Could that affect breastfeeding?

Yes. Any breast surgery or breast injury can affect breastfeeding. Everyone's body is different, and it's impossible to know whether the surgery will impact breastfeeding. It may. It may not. Having frequent weight checks is one way to know that your baby is thriving on your milk.

Breast Augmentation/Implants

Many women with breast implants have happy breast-feeding experiences. However, mothers with implants may have more problems with low milk supply than women without implants. Breastfeeding will not harm the implants.

One problem is that the implant itself takes up milk storage space inside the breast and may tell the milk cells to make less milk. Another problem is possible damage to the nerves and ducts that resulted from the surgery. If the surgical incision was around the areola, there are more potential milk supply issues. It's important to have weekly or more frequent weight checks of the baby for at least the 1st month.

Engorgement and tight bras can further decrease milk supply. Use tank tops with shelf bras for the 1st week or 2 to avoid pressure against the breast.

If you feel more comfortable, talk about your surgery when you're alone with your healthcare provider, when your partner or family is not present.

Breast Reduction Surgery

Women who have had breast reduction surgery have a greater chance of not making enough milk and stop breastfeeding sooner than women who have not. Here are some questions to ask yourself and to discuss with your healthcare provider and your baby's healthcare provider:

- Do you have sensation in your breasts, especially around your nipples?
- Can milk flow through the breast to the nipple?

- Can milk flow through the nipple pores?
- Did you notice breast changes during pregnancy?

Some mothers who have had breast reduction surgery experience difficulty with milk supply. Some mothers find that they feel milk in their breast, but because of the surgery, the milk can't get out of the breast. If you're having problems, ask a breastfeeding care provider to observe a nursing and do before-and-after weights to confirm that you have adequate milk transfer. Inform your healthcare provider and the baby's healthcare provider about your past surgery, and make sure the baby is examined regularly for adequate nutrition. Some mothers with breast reduction surgery use an at-breast supplementer.

Other Breast Surgery

Any breast or chest surgery or injury could negatively impact breastfeeding. The only way to know is to breastfeed and receive follow-up care from healthcare providers. Tell your healthcare provider and your baby's healthcare provider about your surgery.

Any breast surgery or injury could negatively impact breast-feeding.

169

PART SEVEN

Special Situations

My baby was born early.
How do I provide milk for my baby?

I'm pregnant with more than one baby.
Can I breastfeed?

My baby was born with a birth defect.
Can I breastfeed?

More ...

88. I've been told to stop breastfeeding because of a newly diagnosed medical problem. What should I do?

This sometimes happens. When a medical condition is diagnosed, a new drug is prescribed, a diagnostic procedure (such as an X-ray or nuclear diagnostic procedure, MRI, or CT scan) is ordered, or a dental procedure is needed, mothers and their healthcare providers wonder about the risk. Will the drug go through the milk to the baby? Will the drug affect the milk supply? Will the procedure affect the milk? Will anything harmful linger in the mother's body and her milk?

You have your entire pregnancy to research the drugs you routinely take and to find out about the safety of the drugs during breastfeeding (remember that breastfeeding and pregnancy are different, however; drugs that aren't safe in pregnancy may be fine during breastfeeding). But when the problem develops suddenly during breastfeeding, it's more urgent for you to research and consider the possibilities.

Mara, a 32-year-old woman who gave birth to a daughter 8 years ago, had planned to breastfeed. Unfortunately, she had an emergency hysterectomy immediately after the birth. When she left the hospital, she was taking a new prescription drug to lower her blood pressure. She doesn't remember anyone telling her that she could breastfeed, so she just assumed that she couldn't because she no longer had a uterus and was taking a new prescription drug. So Mara fed her baby formula and was full of sadness and regrets about her lost breastfeeding experience. Eight years later she learned that the blood-pressure-lowering drug was considered safe for breastfeeding mothers and that it's OK to breastfeed after a hysterectomy.

Special Situations

173

Mara didn't discuss breastfeeding with her healthcare providers, and they didn't bring up the subject with her. It's important to remind every healthcare provider that breastfeeding is important to you.

Get up-to-date information about drugs and procedures from resources dedicated to lactation and drugs or procedures. There are Internet resources and reference books specifically developed to help women and their healthcare providers consider all the drug and procedure alternatives. See the Appendix for some resources.

89. My baby spits up a lot. Can breastfed babies have reflux?

Both breastfed and formula-fed babies can have reflux. Some amount of spit-up is normal, but spit-up or vomiting that clears the chin can be quite worrisome for mothers and healthcare providers, especially if the baby isn't gaining enough weight. Always talk to your baby's healthcare provider. That person may prescribe reflux medication.

Sometimes breastfed babies spit up because they have nursed very quickly and transferred a lot of milk. By nursing in the Australian or semireclining postures, gravity slows down the flow of milk, making it more manageable for the baby (See Question 21). Be sure not to apply pressure to the back of the baby's head.

90. My baby was born early. How do I provide milk for my baby?

Your prematurely born baby will especially benefit from receiving your milk. Prematurely born babies who receive human milk have faster brain stem maturation. This means that many of the activities that are important—breathing and maintaining body temperature, for example—happen earlier for those premature babies who are fed mother's milk. In addition, such babies have been shown to have a higher IQ, spend fewer days in the hospital, and have fewer complications of prematurity.

Although your baby may be fed intravenously for a while, you will want to start expressing milk as soon as you're able, hopefully within 6 hours of the birth, and then frequently, at least eight times a day using a double-sided electric pump designed for mothers who are pump dependent or by hand expression. Usually, the hospital staff will give you a pumping log to record your expressions. They will also give you specific information about what they want your milk to be expressed into and how they want it labeled and stored. Please follow those directions. For general information on expression and storage of milk, see Questions 39 and 41.

When prematurely born babies are fed mother's milk, the first feedings may be through a tube that goes to the stomach. This feeding tube is often threaded through the nose and changed every day. Small amounts of your colostrum will be sent through the tube to begin protecting your baby from organisms in the environment, to encourage the intestines to grow thicker and stronger, and to begin colonizing the intestines with lactobacillus, the friendly intestinal bacteria promoted by breast milk.

Holding your baby skin to skin with your body in an upright posture is called "kangaroo mother care" or KMC. Babies held this way are warmed by the mother's breasts, hear her comforting heartbeat, and smell her familiar odor. The result? The baby is warmer than in the incubator and experiences less stress. In addition, the mother expresses more milk and has a more optimal breastfeeding experience.

When the baby is ready to receive feedings by mouth, tube feeding usually continues until the baby is able to take all the milk by mouth. Bottle feeding takes more energy and is more stressful than breastfeeding for preemies. (They have lower blood oxygen saturation levels when being bottle fed compared to when being breastfed.) Many newborn intensive care units cup-feed babies when they're separated from their mother because research indicates that it's a safe and effective alternative to the bottle.

At first, many prematurely born babies take longer to transfer milk at the breast compared to full-term infants. Their mouths are small, and they tire easily. Having the opportunity to practice breastfeeding, not the baby's age or size, is what makes all the difference. The more opportunities the baby has to practice, the faster he will learn the skill.

There are community resources to help you breastfeed after you bring your baby home from the hospital. Please see Question 18 for more information on breastfeeding support.

91. I'm pregnant with more than one baby. Can I breastfeed?

Yes. Mothers have successfully provided breast milk for and breastfed twins, triplets, quads, and other high-order multiples. You may think at first that it would be easier to feed formula so that other people could help with the feedings, but mothers have told us how much they enjoy having special time with their babies, doing something only they can do.

Women can definitely make milk for more than one baby. Remember that milk removal and suckling are the messages that are relayed to the milk-making system. Mothers who nurse multiple babies have more milk removal and suckling stimulation than those who are breastfeeding one and so should expect that the milk-making system is getting more messages than a mother nursing one baby.

92. I'm breastfeeding multiples. How will I make enough milk for my babies?

There are several strategies that increase the amount of milk in mothers of multiples:

- Begin expressing or breastfeeding as soon as possible after the babies are born, hopefully within 6 hours after the birth.
- Breastfeed or express milk 10–12 times a day.
- For maximum milk collection, collect milk from both breasts simultaneously when pumping or hand expressing.
- If using a breast pump, use one that is designed for pump-dependent mothers. Be sure that it's working properly. Use a double collecting kit. Be sure the flange is the right size for you. Does your nipple move freely during the entire pumping session? If not, you need a larger flange.
- Work toward breastfeeding two babies at the same time for increased milk production.

- If one baby is more vigorous, nurse that baby at the same time as a less vigorous one. That way, the more vigorous baby will drive the **milk ejection reflex** (or **letdown reflex**) in both breasts.
- If you have more than two babies, consider a rotation strategy. For example, a mother of triplets might nurse triplets 1 and 2 simultaneously and then nurse triplet 3 on both breasts. At the next nursing, she might breastfeed triplets 2 and 3 together and then triplet 1 on both breasts. Then at the next feeding, she might breastfeed triplets 3 and 1 together and triplet 2 on both breasts. (See Figures 30–35 for ways that you can position two babies for simultaneous breastfeeding.)
- Mothers of quads usually rotate pairs. Quad 1 and 2 nurse together first at a feeding. Quads 3 and 4 nurse last. At the next feeding, quads 3 and 4 nurse first, and quads 1 and 2 nurse last.

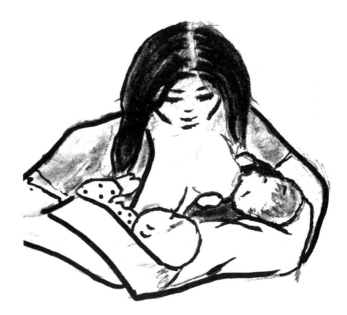

Figure 30 Breastfeeding Twins (a)
Both babies are in the "football" position.

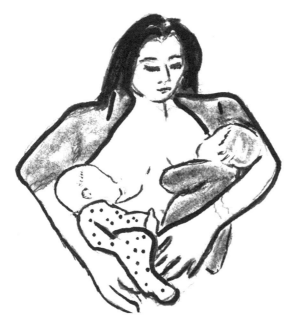

Figure 31   Breastfeeding Twins (b)
The mother is in a semireclining posture and the babies are positioned along the length of her body.

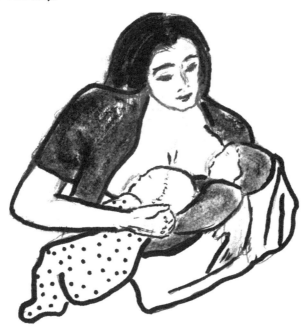

Figure 32   Breastfeeding Twins (c)
Both babies are in the "cradle" position.

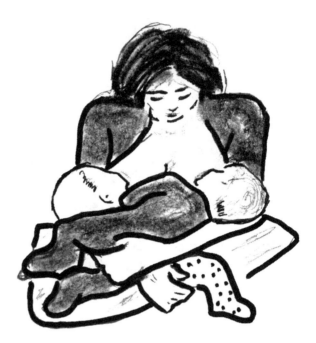

Figure 33   Breastfeeding Twins (d)
The mother is in a sitting posture and the babies are crossed over each other's body.

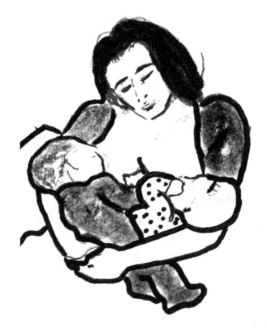

Figure 34   Breastfeeding Twins (e)
The mother is in a semireclining posture and the babies are crossed over each other's body.

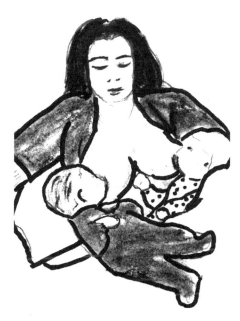

Figure 35   Breastfeeding Twins (f)
The mother uses pillows to support the babies so that her hands are free.

Nursing multiple babies may seem challenging. Don't worry—multiple birth babies learn patience at an early age!

93. My baby was born with a birth injury. Can that interfere with breastfeeding?

Yes. But babies, even babies who can't breastfeed, can still get expressed breast milk from their mothers. Many birth injuries resolve in days or weeks. Until that time, your baby can get your milk, and you keep open the possibility of breastfeeding your baby.

Many birth injuries resolve in days or weeks.

Birth injuries and other conditions can make breastfeeding more difficult. Some problems are visible and diagnosed before the first breastfeeding after birth. Sometimes babies with injuries and other conditions are in pain and cry when moved or held. Problems with breastfeeding often lead to further medical investigation, when the condition is discovered. Torticollis, where the neck muscles are shorter on one side than the other; hematoma, where the head has been impacted; and brachial plexus injury, where the baby is in a great deal of pain when moved are a few of the conditions that challenge positioning the baby at the breast. Any visible problem can be complicated by a swallowing disorder, although babies can have a swallowing disorder without any other condition.

If your baby has a condition that makes being at the breast uncomfortable, experiment with a variety of postures and positions, and breastfeed in a way that makes the baby comfortable. It may be best to rotate your body, rather than the baby, so that the baby can nurse on the second breast.

Speech and language pathologists, occupational therapists, and physical therapists are among the healthcare professionals who can evaluate your baby's capabilities and suggest exercises and feeding strategies. Ask your baby's physician about resources available in your community and possible referrals. Special imaging techniques can evaluate a baby's swallow and may suggest positions and techniques to improve your baby's feeding skills.

Even if your baby cannot breastfeed today, breast milk is the ideal choice for your baby.

94. My baby was born with a birth defect. Can I breastfeed?

That depends on the type of birth defect, the extent of the problem, the baby's medical condition, and the supportive treatments your baby is getting that may influence her ability to feed at the breast. Even if your baby can't breastfeed today, expressed breast milk may be an important part of her diet.

Josie's son, Ricky, was born with Pierre Robin Sequence, a complex birth defect that impacts the ability to breastfeed because of a shortened jaw, recessed chin, and palate cleft—among other problems, such as respiratory distress. Multiple surgeries were planned, and breastfeeding was impossible because the baby could not nurse and breathe at the same time. Josie expressed her milk using an electric breast pump for 7 months. Ricky's doctors told Josie that her milk helped protect Ricky from colds and ear infections. Because he was so healthy, he had surgery earlier.

95. I'm pregnant and was told my baby may have Down syndrome. Should I give up my plan to breastfeed?

Breast milk and breastfeeding may be even more important to a baby who is born with Down syndrome because children with the condition experience obesity, diabetes, and cardiac problems in higher frequency. In addition, breastfeeding may encourage tongue motions that aid children with Down syndrome in speaking more clearly. Breast milk is easily digested and may contribute to improved learning ability.

How to Get Breastfeeding off to a Good Start for a Baby with Down Syndrome

- Hold your baby skin to skin as soon as possible after you give birth and as much as possible after that.
- Keep your baby close by you. A sling is ideal.
- Express milk within 6 hours after your baby is born, and express after each nursing for the first several weeks to be sure that your body makes enough milk.
- Use a pump that is designed for continual, not casual, use—or learn the technique of hand expression.
- Feed your baby at least every hour and a half. Babies with Down syndrome may not demonstrate feeding cues, or the cues may be very subtle, especially at first.
- Have your breastfeedings assessed by a breastfeeding care provider. Before-and-after feeding weights will help you know how much your baby is transferring and whether you should supplement with your expressed breast milk. Consider an at-breast feeder to supplement rather than a bottle. Babies with Down syndrome seem to be easily imprinted on bottle nipples and may have problems going back and forth between the bottle and the breast.
- Try expressing a small amount of milk just before putting the baby to your breast so that the milk is already flowing. You may have to hold the baby at your breast and support your breast during the feeding. If the baby seems to sleep and stops suckling, try alternate massage (i.e., breast compression), which is described in Question 24.
- Go to all the recommended pediatric appointments. Babies with Down syndrome gain weight more slowly than other children, whether breastfed or formula fed.
- Ask your pediatrician and other families with Down syndrome about community resources to improve

your baby's ability to feed. Speech and language pathologists, speech therapists, and occupational therapists can help you by evaluating your baby's abilities and teach you helpful exercises to improve feeding at the breast.

96. My baby has a cleft lip and palate. I need suggestions for breastfeeding. Are there special techniques that might help?

Clefts differ in their configuration and how they may impact breastfeeding. Babies can have a **cleft lip**—with either a single (unilateral) cleft of the upper lip or a double (bilateral) cleft of the upper lip. They can also have a single (unilateral) palate cleft or a double (bilateral) palate cleft, which affects both sides of the palate. There are also clefts that affect both the upper lip *and* the palate. These can be unilateral or bilateral.

Surgery will not only change your baby's appearance; it will affect your feeding strategies. Your healthcare team will give you individualized information about your baby's surgery schedule, but babies can continue to receive their mother's milk after the surgery. And breastfeeding as soon as the baby is out of recovery has been shown to be safe and to enhance the baby's growth.

Many babies with clefts, especially cleft lip and unilateral palate cleft, are able to breastfeed right after birth. Maximizing your milk supply by expressing after feeding is always recommended for the first weeks. Also, feedings tend to be longer for babies with clefts because these babies have more of a "piston," or chewing, action at the breast rather than the efficient "rocker" motion.

Clefts differ in their configuration and how they may impact breastfeeding.

Cleft lip

a congenital birth defect causing a division or split in the lip

For Cleft Lip without Palatal Involvement

The function of a baby's upper lip is to form a seal against the breast so that the vacuum (i.e., negative pressure) created draws the nipple deeply into the baby's mouth. If your baby has cleft lip, your breast can fill the cleft area. The breast should be soft (hand expression just before feeding may make the breast more pliable). Putting a rolled facecloth under the breast may help lift it up and make the seal.

Some mothers use their thumb or finger to move the sides of the cleft together, forming the seal.

Most mothers find that they need to do alternate massage (breast compression) to increase milk transfer. Alternate massage is described in Question 24.

For Cleft Palate

With a one-sided (unilateral) cleft, you can position your breast on an angle so that the breast tissue covers the cleft and creates a vacuum inside the baby's mouth. Usually, it's best if you position the baby so that the cleft side is down; that way, gravity helps as well. Don't turn the baby over when you move the baby to the other side, just slide the baby over as in Figure 29.

If the cleft is large, or bilateral, your breast may not cover the missing area. In this case you may use an obturator. In the past obturators fell out of favor because they were stiff and the baby had to be anesthetized to be fitted for one. Now obturators are made out of the same material as athletic mouth guards, and the fitting takes only a few minutes—with the baby awake. Obturators are inexpensive, and can be fitted and remade as the baby grows.

Your breastfeeding helper may suggest that you use a nipple shield, a thin latex cover for your breast that covers the baby's palate when your breast is positioned in the baby's mouth. If supplementation is needed, you can insert an at-breast feeder tube inside the nipple shield, and the baby can receive all feedings at the breast.

For Unilateral Cleft Lip and Palate

If you put your breast into the baby's mouth on an angle, with your nipple pointed toward the intact area of the palate, your breast can make a seal in the lip area and cover the palate area. Using alternate massage (breast compression) may increase the amount of milk transfer.

97. Can I bring back my milk supply? I stopped nursing and want to start again.

There are two issues here: the milk supply and the baby feeding at the breast. The possibility of bringing back your milk supply depends on several factors:

- Why did you stop breastfeeding? If you stopped because you were struggling with your milk supply, you need to determine the problem and whether it can be fixed.

Celine struggled with breastfeeding her new baby daughter, Maura. Three-year-old twins plus a 5-year-old took a lot of her time and energy and Maura was an easy baby right from the beginning. In addition, Celine was a home day care provider and had an additional five children to care for during working hours.

In the hospital Celine supplemented Maura with the same formula she had given the twins. Within days of leaving the hospital, Maura was entirely formula fed and she began spitting up. As the days went by, the spitting up became worse and worse. Maura also cried and fussed for hours each day.

Celine wondered whether changing formula might solve the problem or even whether going back to breastfeeding was possible. The nurse at the pediatrician's office helped Celine build up her milk supply. After 2 weeks she exclusively breastfed Maura.

- How long has it been since you had milk? How long has it been since you gave birth? The closer mothers are to giving birth or to making milk, the faster the supply comes back.
- How long has it been since the baby breastfed? How old is the baby? Was the baby ever breastfed? Young babies who have breastfed recently may go back to the breast and remember how to remove milk effectively and efficiently, but a baby who is several weeks old and has never breastfed can be more challenging. Babies over 4 months old may be distracted at the breast (see Question 69) even if they have been consistently breastfed, so returning to breastfeeding after stopping may be more difficult for them.

A breastfeeding care provider can give you individualized counseling about your situation. In general, we start mothers expressing milk and replacing formula with expressed milk as one part of the strategy, and we think about breastfeeding as a separate strategy for which an at-breast feeder might be needed as a temporary measure.

In emergency situations, such as hurricanes or other disasters, mothers should be encouraged to breastfeed and express milk. Women have breastfed in unimaginable conditions. Mother's milk provides the baby with protection against disease and exposure to any harmful organisms in contaminated water. Mothers make breast milk even when their diet is less than ideal, so breastfeeding is possible even when mothers have little or no food.

98. Can I breastfeed without giving birth to a baby?

Yes, you can—because women's breasts develop during the time they're in their mother's womb and then as they reach physical maturity. Pregnancy continues the development, so women who have been pregnant or have had a miscarriage have milk-making cells that are more ready to make milk. But women who have never been pregnant have produced milk, too.

Technologies such as at-breast feeders, breast pumps, and hormone therapy can help women produce milk and breastfeed for a baby they have not given birth to. But at this point in time, we do not know which strategies are best. As a result, women often do everything they can to promote milk production, including working with their physician to use progestin-type hormones to simulate a pregnancy, pumping to simulate a baby nursing, and using an at-breast feeding system to experience breastfeeding.

Talk over your individual situation and plans with your breastfeeding care provider. That way, he or she can direct you to resources and more specific information for you.

99. I heard something on TV about milk banks and women using milk from other mothers to feed their babies. What is a milk bank, and how does one work?

According to Lois D. W. Arnold, PhD, an international expert on milk and milk banking and the chair of the National Commission on Donor Milk Banking of the American Breastfeeding Institute: Milk banks were established in the United States and in Europe in the early 1900s. Milk from women who were healthy was used to feed hospitalized premature and ill babies. In Boston, the Children's Floating Hospital used the milk collected to treat "summer diarrheal disease." Such establishments screened their donors carefully for illness, and many milk banks even inspected the homes of the donors for cleanliness. Milk was tested for quality and was pasteurized to ensure that babies receiving the milk would not get even sicker.

These principles remain in effect today. *Guidelines for the Establishment and Operation of a Donor Human Milk Bank* have been developed by the Human Milk Banking Association of North America (HMBANA). These guidelines were developed in consultation with various government agencies, infectious disease experts, and healthcare providers. These guidelines are reviewed and revised regularly. Nonprofit donor milk banks in the United States and Canada that are members of HMBANA all operate according to these guidelines to ensure the safety and quality of the donor milk when it's dispensed.

Donors must be thoroughly screened for health, including blood tests for **HIV**, hepatitis B and C, human

T-cell leukemia virus, and syphilis. All milk is pasteurized (heat treated) before distribution to kill any bacteria or viruses that may be present. This pasteurization does decrease the milk's anti-infective properties somewhat, but not entirely. Nutritional properties of human milk are largely heat stable.

I'll be going back to work. Could I get some milk for my baby?

Banked donor human milk from a HMBANA milk bank is a prescribed item and is used for premature and sick infants and children. Occasionally, sick adults also require donor milk. Donor milk is not dispensed for reasons other than a baby's or mother's medical/ nutritional condition. Therefore, a physician must write an order for donor milk.

In some cases in the United States, health insurance covers prescribed donor milk. In other countries social security covers access to donor milk, and parents don't have to pay a processing fee for the milk. In the United States a processing fee is charged per ounce of milk. This fee is not a charge for the milk, but a means of covering some of the overhead costs involved in screening donors and processing the milk.

Donor milk seems expensive. Could I get milk through another arrangement?

Wet nurses exist still in many parts of the world. These are women who nurse someone else's baby for a fee. This is strongly discouraged in the United States because of the lack of donor screening and the inability to ensure the milk's safety.

HIV
a group of retro-viruses that infect and destroy helper T cells of the immune system—also called "AIDS virus" and "human immuno-deficiency virus"

Special Situations

A physician must write an order for donor milk.

Many women who don't know about donor human milk banks may think about borrowing milk from a relative or a neighbor. This also isn't a safe practice because relatives and friends may keep secrets from each other and not disclose risky sexual behavior. They may also not know that an illness or condition they have may be a risk for a baby who is not their own biologic baby. For example, the herpes virus can be transmitted through human milk if a breastfeeding mother has a herpes lesion on her breast or nipple. Do you always know when your friends or relatives have herpes? No. And even if you heat the milk to get rid of the herpes virus, it's not adequate to ensure the milk's safety.

Some women have been known to nurse each other's babies when they share babysitting arrangements. This situation is also unsafe for the same reasons.

What about buying milk over the Internet? I've seen it posted on eBay.

This is even more dangerous because the milk may have been tampered with in some way, with the potential to cause even greater harm to the recipient. People may dilute the milk to increase the number of ounces they sell, thereby making more money for themselves, but compromising the nutrition of the infant. Someone may even sell cow's milk or goat's milk, passing it off as human milk. There's no way for a buyer to know this, and it could endanger a baby with a severe cow's milk protein allergy. There's also no way of guaranteeing that the milk is safe from a bacteriologic or viral standpoint.

Although there's no federal legislation that restricts this practice, the buyer should beware! In the United

States, only California and New York have legislation that regulates donor human milk banking and makes it illegal to purchase or donate milk without using a milk bank that is licensed to operate in those states. These licensed milk banks operate as tissue banks and are subject to regulation and inspection to ensure that standards are maintained and recipients will be safe.

The convenient and safe way to acquire human milk is to get it through a HMBANA-member milk bank. The locations of HMBANA milk banks are available at http://www.hmbana.org.

What if I want to become a donor?

Women with excess amounts of milk who are healthy are welcomed as donors. After finding the closest milk bank (not every state has one), you can make a phone call and begin the screening process. Some milk banks accept out-of-state donors and cover the costs of shipping milk to them. Ongoing donors are instructed in how to collect their milk and minimize contamination, and they collect milk in containers provided by the milk bank, delivering or shipping the frozen milk when they have collected enough for a batch. Sometimes milk banks will also accept milk that has been previously collected, especially in amounts exceeding several hundred ounces.

It's worth noting that donating milk can be a therapeutic part of the grieving process when a mother loses a baby or gives one up for adoption. The Mothers' Milk Bank in Indianapolis, Indiana, has grant funds for a bereavement program that involves donating milk previously collected for a sick or premature infant.

100. Where can I get more information about breastfeeding?

Ask your own healthcare provider or your baby's healthcare provider.

For technical questions about breastfeeding, you may want to contact a breastfeeding care provider in your area. This person should be able to help you with individualized care or direct you to other resources. See Question 18 for more information about how to find a breastfeeding care provider. More information about organizations that train and certify breastfeeding care providers can be found in the Appendix.

A list of organizations and Web sites that provide information about breastfeeding can also be found in the Appendix.

Perhaps you have questions about mothering and breastfeeding. La Leche League leaders and other nursing mothers' support group leaders can help with these questions. See the Appendix list for information about contacting La Leche League International.

Every question is important. We encourage you to continue seeking answers to your questions.

Appendix

Books

Hale, T. W. (2006). *Medications and mother's milk* (12th ed.). Amarillo, TX: Hale.

Hale, T. W., & G. A. McAfee. (2005). *Medication guide for breastfeeding moms*. Amarillo, TX: Pharmasoft.

Kendall-Tackett, K. A. (2005). *The hidden feelings of motherhood* (2nd ed.). Amarillo, TX: Pharmasoft.

La Leche League International. (2004). *The womanly art of breastfeeding* (7th ed.). New York: Plume.

Breastfeeding Clothing

Bravado! Designs
http://www.bravadodesigns.com
By telephone: 800-590-7802

LactationConnection.com
http://www.lactationconnection.com
By telephone: 800-216-8151

La Leche League International
http://www.lalecheleague.org
By telephone: 847-519-7730

Motherwear
http://www.motherwear.com
By telephone: 800-950-2500

Breastfeeding Resources

American Academy of Pediatrics
http://www.aap.org
AAP publishes policy statements on breastfeeding such
as:
- Breastfeeding and the Use of Human Milk (2005)
- The Transfer of Drugs and Other Chemicals into
  Human Milk (2001)

Centers for Disease Control and Prevention
http://www.cdc.gov/breastfeeding
By telephone: 800-311-3435
CDC provides information about breastfeeding and
disease, as well as other health-related aspects of
breastfeeding.

Food and Drug Administration (FDA)
http://www.fda.gov/cdrh/breastpumps
The FDA provides resources on milk expression,
breast pumping, and milk storage.

Human Milk Banking Association of North America
(HMBANA)
http://www.hmbana.org
By telephone: 919-861-4530, ext. 226
HMBANA provides referrals to member milk banks
for milk-donating purposes, as well as details about
how to obtain human milk for a sick baby.

International Lactation Consultant Association (ILCA)
http://www.ilca.org
By telephone: 919-861-5577
ILCA provides a referral database of lactation
consultants.

La Leche League International (LLLI)
http://www.lalecheleague.org
By telephone: 847-519-7730
LLLI refers women to leaders of local meetings and
provides helpful documents, books, breastfeeding
equipment, and other resources.

National Library of Medicine—LactMed
http://toxnet.nlm.nih.gov/cgi-bin/sis/htmlgen?LACT
LactMed is a searchable online database of the effects
of medications on breastfeeding babies.

National Women's Health Information Center, US
Department of Health and Human Services, Office
on Women's Health
http://www.womenshealth.gov
By telephone: 800-994-0662
This center provides online information as well as telephone counseling on a variety of women's health
topics, including breastfeeding.

United States Breastfeeding Committee
http://www.usbreastfeeding.org
USBC provides white papers on topics such as
workplace breastfeeding support and breastfeeding
legislation.

US Department of Agriculture, Food, and Nutrition
Service
http://www.fns.usda.gov

This agency administers the Special Supplemental Nutrition Program for Women, Infants, and Children, which provides nutrition and breastfeeding counseling to eligible women and children.

Organizations That Certify Breastfeeding Care Providers

The Academy of Lactation Policy & Practice (ALPP)
http://www.talpp.org
By telephone: 508-833-1500
ALPP certifies lactation counselors.

The International Board of Lactation Consultant Examiners (IBLCE)
http://www.iblce.org
By telephone: 703-560-7330
IBLCE certifies lactation consultants.

Breastfeeding Legislation (United States)

http://maloney.house.gov (search "breastfeeding")
http://usbreastfeeding.org/Issue-Papers/State-Legislation-2004.pdf
http://www.lalecheleague.org (search "breastfeeding legislation")

Breast Milk Storage Containers

LactationConnection.com
http://www.lactationconnection.com
By telephone: 800-216-8151

Mother's Milkmate
http://www.mothersmilkmate.com
By telephone: 800-499-3506

Snappies
http://www.snappiescontainers.com
By telephone: 800-772-8871

Many breast pump companies also make storage
   containers.

Breast Pump Company Web Sites

Avent
http://www.aventamerica.com

Bailey Medical
http://www.baileymed.com

BreastPump.com
http://www.breastpump.com

Hollister
http://www.hollister.com/us

Medela Pumps
http://www.medela.com

Whisper Wear
http://www.whisperwear.com

Whittlestone
http://www.whittlestone.com

Breast Pump Parts

Breast Pump Companies (see Breast Pump Company
   Web Sites)

LactationConnection.com
www.lactationconnection.com
By telephone: 800-216-8151

Feeding Supplies

Lact-Aid
http://www.lact-aid.com

LactationConnection.com
http://www.lactationconnection.com
By telephone: 800-216-8151

Medela
http://www.medela.com

Glossary

allergy: an abnormal reaction to a protein that is eaten, inhaled, or otherwise encountered

anemia: a condition in which the blood is deficient in red blood cells, in hemoglobin, or in total volume; typically refers to iron-deficiency anemia

areola: the darkened area around the nipple

asthma: an inflammation or swelling of the airway, leading to breathing difficulty, wheezing, and coughing

Baby-Friendly Hospital Initiative (BFHI): a United Nations Children's Fund and World Health Organization program recognizing hospitals and birth centers that implement the "Ten Steps to Successful Breastfeeding"

bilirubin: a by-product of the breakdown of the hemoglobin portion of red blood cells

carbohydrates: the chemical name for sugars, starches, and cellulose

central nervous system: the brain and the spinal cord

cleft lip: a congenital birth defect causing a division or split in the lip

cleft palate: a congenital birth defect causing a division or opening in the roof of the mouth

colostrum: the first milk, produced in the breasts by the 5th month of pregnancy—colostrum is thick, sticky, and clear to yellowish in color; is high in protein and vitamin A; causes a laxative effect, helping the baby pass meconium; and contains immunoglobulins (mostly IgA), which protect the baby from infections

complementary food: food other than breast milk that complements, but does not replace, breastfeeding

congenital: a condition that has existed from birth

contaminants: factors that make a product unclean or impure

cradle posture: a breastfeeding position in which the mother holds the baby on her lap with his head resting on her forearm directly in front of the breast (aka "Madonna posture")

crib death: the unexpected and sudden death, of unknown origin, of a seemingly normal and healthy infant that occurs during sleep; also called "sudden infant death syndrome," or SIDS

cross-cradle posture: a breastfeeding position in which the mother holds the baby on her lap with his head resting on her forearm of the arm opposite the suckled breast; the hand of her arm on the same side either supports the breast or is free

dehydration: a condition in which the infant is not receiving adequate fluids or is unable to maintain adequate hydration because of a metabolic reason; symptoms of this potentially serious problem include lethargy (extreme fatigue and weakness), sunken eyes, a sunken soft spot on the infant's head, and little or no urine

docosahexaenoic acid (DHA): a long-chain polyunsaturated fatty acid believed to support an infant's rapidly developing nervous system

Down syndrome: a congenital condition characterized by moderate to severe mental retardation, also called "Down's" or "trisomy 21"

doula: an individual who supports the mother during the perinatal period, colloquially known as "mothering the mother"

eczema: a noncontagious skin inflammation, characterized chiefly by redness, itching, and the outbreak of lesions that may become encrusted and scaly

engorgement: swelling in the breast that blocks milk flow, caused by inadequate or infrequent milk removal; the breast will be hot and painful and will look tight and shiny; with severe engorgement, milk production may stop

exclusive breastfeeding: when a baby is given no drinks or foods other than breast milk and no pacifiers or artificial nipples

football or clutch posture: a breastfeeding posture in which the baby is tucked under the mother's arm, with baby's feet behind his mother's back and the baby's shoulders supported in the palm of her hand

foremilk: the milk present in the breast at the beginning of a breastfeed

formula: a food made from cow's milk or soy milk that has been chemically altered to make it appropriate for the nutrition of human babies

galactosemia: a rare congenital inability of the body to metabolize the simple sugar galactose, causing damage to the liver, central nervous system, and other body systems

gastrointestinal: having to do with the stomach and intestinal tract

HIV: a group of retroviruses that infect and destroy helper T cells of the immune system—also called "AIDS virus" and "human immunodeficiency virus"

hyperbilirubinemia: high levels of bilirubin in the blood

hypoglycemia: low blood sugar

immunoglobulins: proteins that provide immunity

inflammation: a localized reaction of tissue to the presence of items perceived to be foreign or another irritation, injury, or infection that is characterized by pain, redness, and swelling

inverted nipple: a nipple that turns inward when stimulated

jaundice: a condition that results when red blood cells break down faster than the liver can handle, yellowing the skin; in the newborn, normal physiologic jaundice is caused by the immaturity of the liver

lactic acid: the breakdown product of energy stored in the muscles that is released during intense exercise, such as sprinting

lactose: a sugar found only in mammalian milk

lactose intolerance: a condition occurring in some adults in which the body does not produce adequate amounts of lactase, causing abdominal bloating, gas, and pain when foods containing lactose are consumed

letdown reflex: the milk ejection reflex, the spontaneous ejection of milk from the breast

lochia: the discharge from the uterus after birth

Madonna posture: a breastfeeding posture in which the mother holds the baby on her lap with his head resting on the mother's forearm directly in front of the breast (aka "cradle posture")

malnutrition: refers to those who are either overfed, underfed, or unable to correctly use the food they're receiving

mastitis: inflammation in the breast causing localized tenderness, redness, and heat; mothers with mastitis may have a fever or headache and may feel tired, achy, or nauseous; mastitis may or may not be caused by an infection

meconium: the first stool of a newborn, varying from greenish black to light brown with a tarry consistency

milk duct: the narrow tube structure that carries milk to the nipple

milk ejection reflex: a reflex initiated by the production of the hormone oxytocin, which causes the milk to flow

Montgomery glands: the small glands of the darker skin of the breast around the nipple. The Montgomery glands become more noticeable during pregnancy. They produce a sticky, shiny antimicrobial lubricant that coats the breast and nipple

newborn: a human baby younger than 1 month of age

nursing supplementer: fine plastic tubing, with one end attached to a container holding expressed human milk or formula and the other end taped to the breast

oxytocin: the hormone that makes the milk flow in response to nipple stretching and the newborn baby's hands touching the breast. Oxytocin also contracts the uterus in labor and is released during orgasm

prolactin: hormone that stimulates milk production

rooting: natural instinct of the newborn to turn his head toward the nipple and open his mouth when mouth area is gently stroked with the nipple

SIDS: sudden infant death syndrome—see **crib death**

skin-to-skin holding: the practice of holding the infant so that his bare chest is against that of his mother or father (the baby is held under the parent's clothing and covered as needed for warmth); this technique helps the baby regulate heart rate, respiratory rate, and body temperature and facilitates early breastfeeding

sucking: drawing into the mouth by forming a partial vacuum with the lips and tongue

tandem nursing: nursing two children of different pregnancies—for example, a newborn and a toddler

"Ten Steps to Successful Breastfeeding": guidelines developed by the United Nations Children's Fund (UNICEF) and the World Health Or-

ganization (WHO) that protect and promote breastfeeding in facilities that provide maternity services and care for newborn infants—see **Baby-Friendly Hospital Initiative**

type 1 (insulin-dependent) diabetes: a chronic illness caused by insufficient production of insulin and resulting in abnormal metabolism of carbohydrates, fats, and proteins; symptoms include increased sugar levels in the blood and urine, excessive thirst, frequent urination, and unexplained weight loss; this disease is treated with insulin and is also called "insulin-dependent diabetes mellitus"

type 2 (non-insulin-dependent) diabetes: a milder form of diabetes that typically appears first in adulthood and is associated with obesity and an inactive lifestyle; this disease often has no symptoms, is usually diagnosed by tests that indicate glucose intolerance, and is treated with changes in diet, exercise, and medications; it is also called "non-insulin-dependent diabetes mellitus"

Index